PRAISE FOR *THE LDN BOOK*

"As a practicing physician who has used LDN as a cornerstone therapy for over fifteen years, I can say without equivocation that LDN is the most important and successful medicine I have ever used. I often joke that if not for LDN I couldn't pay my mortgage; I've had so many new patients referred to me by someone whose life has improved dramatically through the use of LDN. And despite my knowledge and experience with LDN, I've learned a great deal from *The LDN Book*—aspects of its basic science I hadn't known, new uses, and how its uses can inform us about the causes of various diseases. This is a wonderful book for any patient with an autoimmune disease, cancer, depression, or a host of other conditions and is a *must*-read for any physician whose goal is to help their patients."

—**Dr. Thomas Cowan**, author of *The Fourfold Path to Healing*;
coauthor of *The Nourishing Traditions Book of Baby & Child Care*

"I first came across LDN several years ago when a medical colleague said I should look into its positive effects in patients with MS, Crohn's disease, and other autoimmune disorders. I was so impressed with what I read that I helped submit a petition to the UK government to ask for funding for further research into this inexpensive drug. But, as with so many petitions, no progress was made. I hope *The LDN Book*—which presents up-to-date findings that again confirm the efficacy of this safe, cheap, generic drug in helping to control many chronic, disabling conditions—is read by those in the Department of Health and by all doctors caring for patients with autoimmune disease. In the UK, LDN has been stranded in limbo; maybe now the time has come for it to be accepted as a recognized therapy that could, at least, be tried on those suffering such long-term diseases of the immune system."

—**Dr. Chris Steele**, MBE, general practitioner;
medical presenter on ITV's *This Morning*

"Low Dose Naltrexone (LDN) was discovered by my husband and partner, Dr. Bernard Bihari. Incredibly informative and superbly written by various members of the medical profession sharing their experiences using this extraordinary drug, *The LDN Book* honors his legacy in helping patients suffering from autoimmune and other diseases to regain their health and their lives."

Young

The
LDN
Book

The
LDN
Book

How a Little-Known Generic Drug
— Low Dose Naltrexone —
Could Revolutionize Treatment
for Autoimmune Diseases, Cancer,
Autism, Depression, and More

EDITED BY
Linda Elsegood

Chelsea Green Publishing
White River Junction, Vermont

Project Manager: Alexander Bullett
Developmental Editor: Michael Metivier
Copy Editor: Deborah Heimann
Proofreader: Helen Walden
Indexer: Lee Lawton
Designer: Melissa Jacobson

Printed in the United States of America.
First printing February, 2016.
10 9 8 7 6 5 4 3 2   16 17 18 19 20

Our Commitment to Green Publishing

Chelsea Green sees publishing as a tool for cultural change and ecological stewardship. We strive to align our book manufacturing practices with our editorial mission and to reduce the impact of our business enterprise in the environment. We print our books and catalogs on chlorine-free recycled paper, using vegetable-based inks whenever possible. This book may cost slightly more because it was printed on paper that contains recycled fiber, and we hope you'll agree that it's worth it. Chelsea Green is a member of the Green Press Initiative (www. greenpressinitiative.org), a nonprofit coalition of publishers, manufacturers, and authors working to protect the world's endangered forests and conserve natural resources. *The LDN Book* was printed on paper supplied by Thomson-Shore that contains 100% postconsumer recycled fiber.

Library of Congress Cataloging-in-Publication Data
Names: Elsegood, Linda, 1956- , editor.
Title: The LDN book : how a little-known generic drug, low dose naltrexone, could revolutionize treatment for
    autoimmune diseases, cancer, autism, depression, and more / edited by Linda Elsegood.
Other titles: Low dose naltrexone book
Description: White River Junction, Vermont : Chelsea Green Publishing, [2016]
    | Includes bibliographical references and index.
Identifiers: LCCN 2015041133| ISBN 9781603586641 (pbk.) | ISBN 9781603586658 (ebook)
Subjects: | MESH: Naltrexone—therapeutic use. | Dose-Response Relationship, Drug. | Naltrexone—
    pharmacology. | Narcotic Antagonists—therapeutic use. | Opioid Peptides—metabolism.
Classification: LCC RM328 | NLM QV 89 | DDC 615.1/9—dc23
LC record available at http://lccn.loc.gov/2015041133

Chelsea Green Publishing
85 North Main Street, Suite 120
White River Junction, VT 05001
(802) 295-6300
www.chelseagreen.com

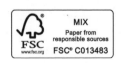

To my late father,
who believed I could achieve anything if I tried hard enough.
Dad, thank you for always supporting me, and
for making me the person I am today!

CONTENTS

PREFACE

As the founder of the LDN Research Trust, I have been in contact with thousands of people from around the world suffering from a multitude of diseases and afflictions. I've also witnessed, through their testimonies, how low dose naltrexone (LDN) has helped ease their symptoms and enabled them to live more enjoyable lives.

My own LDN story began in 1969, when at the age of thirteen I contracted glandular fever, also known as mono. I was seriously ill and away from school for six months. After that, strange things started to happen: trapped nerves here and there, slipped discs; my life seemed to become a never-ending series of health travails.

But things really took a turn for the worse when, in December of 1999, my mother suffered a serious heart attack, the trauma of which affected me badly. I was working full time, commuting two and a half hours to work every day, visiting and caring for my mother and father and, on top of it all, running the family home. I was constantly fatigued.

The following January I came down with a bad flu that kept me home from work for two weeks, and it was followed by a case of gastroenteritis. My immune system was compromised, so it took me at least three additional weeks to recover. This bout of ill health continued when I apparently slipped a disc, causing pins and needles sensations in my right leg. My energy levels were continuing to fall rapidly, I was finding it difficult to cope, and I had to sleep constantly.

At around Easter of that year I decided I had to break this cycle. I took a week off from work and, with my younger daughter, Laura, went to Portugal with the hope that I would start feeling better. Ominously, the day before we left, the left side of my tongue felt burned, as if I'd eaten hot melted cheese, even though I could not remember eating anything like that. Sadly, our vacation sun was nowhere to be seen. Portugal was unbelievably wet, cold, and windy, wind that made the left side of my face numb and tingly.

Back home, I went to see my general practitioner, who thought I had a trapped nerve in my neck. He said I should see a neurologist. However, the earliest available appointment was not for another four months. When the appointment came, my neurologist debated whether I had either had a mild stroke, contracted a foreign disease, developed a brain tumor, or developed multiple sclerosis. Which diagnosis was I meant to hope for? I just wanted him to give me a pill and send me on my way.

Things got worse over the next few weeks. I frequently lost my balance, and the left side of my face, head, tongue, and nose became completely numb with the now familiar feeling of pins and needles. When trying to stand up I either fainted or fell over. Every day I seemed to lose some ability, starting with the hearing in my left ear. The pains and fog in my head were terrible, and I started having double vision. I slept twenty hours a day, which was the only saving grace, as when I was asleep I felt nothing.

My doctor prescribed a three-day course of intravenous (IV) steroids; however, these did nothing to help. The steroids caused my face to balloon until I didn't recognize myself anymore; I was flushed red and looked like a beach ball! I then had an MRI scan, a lumbar puncture, and twenty-eight blood tests. I developed optic neuritis, which was incredibly painful. It was at this point that it was feared I might lose my sight and hearing. Six weeks later, I was given another course of IV steroids and began to feel a little better. Multiple sclerosis (MS) was then diagnosed.

I spent the next year mainly in bed. I was having an attack, or exacerbation, every six months or so. It took months to get over one attack only to have another. I now had no balance and had to "furniture walk." I also suffered from vertigo; if I turned my head too quickly everything would spin. I would stumble over nothing, and my legs behaved like rubber bands. More often than not, I ended up on the floor.

At times I had so much pain in my head that I felt nauseous. Because the pain moved around from one part of my head to another, I often felt as if the doctors didn't believe me. They prescribed strong painkillers, which didn't take the pain away completely but at least made it more bearable, though they also caused extreme nausea.

English became like a second language. Words that once seemed so simple were now lost to me. My sentences were confused and nonsensical. I had to speak very slowly in order to select and arrange the right words, and it made me sound as if I'd had a stroke. It was such a tiring effort, and although I still believed I spoke sense, to others it was just a jumble.

The worst part came when I lost control of my bladder and bowels. I can only describe it as similar to sneezing; I had no control, so when the feeling came it would happen straight away. I couldn't leave the house anymore. I started to use a wheelchair more and more often and even bought an electric scooter. The toilet and the bed became my best friends!

In September of 2003 my elder daughter, Sara, got married, and I doubted whether I could even attend the ceremony. After getting showered and dressed, I had so little energy left that all I wanted to do was go back to bed. Though I struggled, I managed to get there, but I came home as soon as I could, which was hard on our entire family. By October I was falling to pieces, always in the hospital seeing a urologist, gynecologist, or gastroenterologist. At the end of the month, my neurologist said he thought I had "progressed" from the *relapsing and remitting* form of MS to *secondary progressive*. He leaned across the desk and shook my hand before opening the door and saying "There's nothing more that can be done for you." He then showed me out without any plan B. I felt very alone and frightened.

It was after a routine visit from the doctor delivering my painkillers that I reached the end. The helpless look in his eye, which I had seen so many times from others, reduced me to making an extreme decision: I had the tablets and the glass of water he'd left me in my hand, and my husband was at work. I thought that my family would eventually understand, and that they would be able to get on with their lives without me. I felt that I could no longer achieve anything, that I was a failure. It was only when I thought of my fifteen-year-old daughter finding me that I realized I couldn't do that to her. But I also realized that if I was going to remain in this world, I needed to do something different in order to live again.

In between my many bathroom visits I used the computer to research how other people were successfully managing their MS. I knew that I couldn't be the only one out there who was suffering like this. I couldn't be that unique. I read a lot about LDN and spoke to people who were taking it. Although I was worried about taking yet another drug, the people who shared their experiences with it calmly stated that if it wasn't going to do any good, then it certainly wasn't going to do any harm. I stopped taking the Rebif and Provigil I was prescribed and started a special diet plus a regime of vitamins and supplements. I discussed LDN with my general practitioner, but after speaking with the partners of the surgery, she said could not prescribe it for me. However, she did agree to monitor me if I found a doctor who would.

In early December I started LDN, thanks to Dr. Bob Lawrence, and the results were amazing. After only three weeks, the awful fog I'd been living with for so long finally lifted, and my liver tests were returning to normal. My brain had felt like an old, out of tune television set, but no more. I could think clearly again, and I was talking coherently. I went from having my fifteen-year-old daughter feed, clothe, and bathe me to being able to take *her* a glass of orange juice when *she* asked. The caretaking roles were finally reverting back to their natural positions. I carried on improving for the next eighteen months. By Christmas of 2004 I was fully functioning again, and my liver tests were back to normal. I felt like *me*. Okay, a "me" with MS, but that didn't matter.

Now I had to decide, should I simply consider myself to be lucky, or tell other people about my experiences? Of course, I chose to let others know about LDN, and became the founder of the LDN Research Trust, which was established in the United Kingdom as a registered charity in 2004. It is the most exciting thing I have ever done. Having regained my strength and faculties, I am able to devote many hours a week to the Trust, helping people to get LDN prescribed and raising funds and awareness to get it into clinical trials.

The LDN Research Trust is a charity that is run solely by volunteers. Our only payment is the amazing stories of success, which I receive daily from users of LDN, telling us how they have gotten their lives back. Currently the charity has over nineteen thousand members with over twelve thousand supporters (at the time of publication) on Facebook from all around the world. My day-to-day work for the charity includes responding to the numerous e-mails and phone calls I receive with requests for information and advice from both patients and health care professionals. I also produce a bimonthly newsletter that I send to subscribers, which includes LDN user stories and articles on the use of LDN by professionals. I am in contact with thousands of LDN-prescribing doctors and pharmacists around the world, with numbers growing weekly.

Additionally, I have organized a number of conferences on LDN, including one in the United Kingdom and two in the United States, with the next to be held in Orlando, Florida, in February 2016, with an anticipated four hundred delegates. This conference will be live streamed around the world.

I have also made over four hundred videos for our Vimeo channel, where listeners can hear interviews with LDN-prescribing doctors, researchers, pharmacists, and people using LDN for many conditions. These have been of great value not only to users and potential users but also to doctors, nurses, pharmacists, and other clinicians.

Finally, through the LDN Research Trust I have been involved with a number of projects aimed at raising awareness and knowledge about LDN, including the creation and development of an LDN Health Tracker App, which required working with a designer to get the App produced in line with my requirements; raising money for and organizing the production of a documentary on LDN that aired in June, 2015; and raising funds for the upcoming MS/LDN trial led by Dr. Jarred Younger.

Over the past eleven years, I've been asked many times to write a book on LDN, but thought "What do I know about writing a book!" Dr. Mark Shukhman in particular, who wrote, with the help of his daughter, Rebecca, this book's chapter on LDN and depression, repeatedly asked me, "So when are you going to write this LDN book?" Needless to say, working on *The LDN Book* has been one of the most interesting challenges I have undertaken, and one in which Dr. Shukhman was more than happy to participate. I have managed, as the Beatles would have said, "with a little help from my friends."

There have been a few wonderful LDN books written in the past; however, I felt that with all of the latest research, trials, and studies that have happened since they were published, the wealth of updated information contained in this book would be of benefit not only for medical profession-als, but for people like myself wishing to learn more about the drug.

There need to be more double-blind, placebo-controlled trials on LDN. This book presents a way to raise awareness and hopefully encourage people to give generously to help fund further research that would be of great benefit to millions of sick people around the world who are suffering from over 180 conditions (and the list grows longer every year) for which LDN may be of help.

For me, it is thanks to LDN that I have a life again, as well as hope for the future. I've now used LDN for over twelve years. Although I have a progressive disease, I can say with confidence that it has shown no sign of progression. My head is clear, my energy levels are up, and I have greater muscle strength.

LDN is not a miracle drug, and it doesn't necessarily work for everyone, but it's something to try. If others find themselves in the deep, dark place I was in, and perhaps don't feel they have the strength to carry on, I want them to know there may be a way forward. If this book can help change just one life for the better, I will see it as a success. Life should be for living, not just surviving!

LINDA ELSEGOOD
FOUNDER, THE LDN RESEARCH TRUST

INTRODUCTION

I don't remember the exact moment when I first decided to become a doctor (I have been practicing general internal medicine now for many years and have had my own solo practice for the last ten). My cousin tells me that it was my mother's idea. My paternal grandfather was a doctor of internal medicine, and maybe my mother thought it would be nice if I continued the family tradition. Regardless, I received a brand new shiny black stethoscope as a present when I was in first grade. I remember being very excited because it really worked. I would listen to the heart of anyone who would let me. I also remember writing my first essay on why I wanted to become a doctor. My reason was simple: I wanted to help people. Over the past several years, however, I have thought about walking away from medicine many times. In fact, I was sure that I was done before I found out about low dose naltrexone (LDN).

When I was in medical school, I discovered that indeed most of us were there because we wanted to help people, even though I'd been told in response to my essay that, no matter what, one should never write that down as the reason. It was too common of an answer, indicating too much emotion and not enough reason. My peers and I were all focused on patients, studying hard and memorizing all kinds of strange facts, so that if we ever encountered a patient who had a very unusual illness, we would know just what to do. Yet several years into practice, I found that my days were filled with insurance paperwork, phone calls, chart reviews, and a stack of unfinished progress notes that would take me long past sunset every day to complete. I was spending more time at the computer than with patients.

Despite all of this, I can tell you that if I thought I was making a difference in anyone's life or truly helping them get better, it would all have been worth it. But that was not the case. My schedule was filled with patients who had chronic disease and who never got better. Every time they came in they needed more medications. Their numbers never got better, their illnesses never improved, and they never felt better. I know that I have patients who have been with me since the beginning who will argue with me about this, but it's true.

This all changed when I found LDN. At first I was very doubtful, and I wrote my first prescription at the insistence of my seventy-year old patient Marla, who had learned all about LDN from the Internet (doctors generally dread patients who bring in information printed off the Internet; they are second only to patients who happen to have a nurse in the family). When Marla's symptoms improved, I thought it was interesting, but I was too busy with my paperwork to actually delve deeper into LDN. I knew it was being used as an alternative medicine to treat multiple sclerosis (MS), and at the time none of my patients had that illness.

Then, years later, I met Christian. At thirty-two, he was the youngest male patient I had with a serious illness. "Doctor Jill, I've done the research on LDN, and I want to try it out for my symptoms," he said. Christian had an episode of what was basically optic neuritis presenting as double vision. Both his brain MRI report and the report from his spinal tap were consistent with MS. Because this episode of double vision was only a single event, his diagnosis was not yet called MS, and was instead called clinically isolated syndrome. It carried a high probability of turning into MS, and his neuro-ophthalmologist recommended aggressive immunosuppressant therapy.

"I understand the risks, and I'm willing to accept them. My symptoms are already nearly gone, and I want to try LDN first, before taking an immunosuppressant," he said. I had mixed feelings about this idea. I knew his specialist and did not want to step on his feet. In addition, I am not a neurologist, and at that time had no experience whatsoever in treating MS, both facts that I pointed out to my patient. However, I am a big proponent of patient choice, and I was willing to support his choice to decline conventional treatment. I carefully documented in his chart that we had discussed all the risks, contraindications, and alternatives.

I followed Christian very closely, seeing him frequently and documenting as thoroughly as possible everything about his case. I prescribed the LDN exactly according to how other clinicians were prescribing it. Christian's symptoms resolved within about five months of starting treatment, and his MRI reports were slightly improved each time we ran them. In a startling development, the MRI of his brain was read as normal at the two-year mark of treatment. There were no longer signs of any disease at all.

Having been trained in traditional allopathic medicine, I was well aware that this was what would be called an anecdotal case. It was possible that his results could be coincidental and completely unrelated to the treatment. However, a year later, when he was still symptom-free, my curiosity about LDN finally got the better of me. I started doing research into LDN. What I discovered was extremely interesting, and completely changed the way that I thought about LDN. During my medical training I had always assumed that if a treatment was not conventional, with double-blind, placebo-controlled, randomized trials, then it was not a legitimate treatment. I discovered that I was wrong.

When I had first heard about LDN, I had no idea who Dr. Bernard Bihari was or how impressive his credentials were. I had no idea how much information was available about LDN's biochemistry; I found that the cellular pathways were known down to the very receptors involved. Before doing my research, I did not realize that small studies and case reports had already been published.

In the year that I started considering LDN seriously, I attended a conference in Las Vegas put together by the LDN Research Trust. It was fascinating to listen to the many speakers talk about their personal experiences with LDN, and to witness the presentations of many interesting case studies. A good number of the doctors had been prescribing LDN for as long as I had been in practice. But throughout the day a question kept bothering me. If LDN was a legitimately successful treatment, then it seemed to me that all these doctors should have been writing up their findings and getting them published. It was during a conversation with one of the oldest doctors in attendance that I finally realized the answer.

All these doctors were just as busy as I was. The only difference was that they were busy taking care of patients. They did not have time to be writing case reports or conducting trials. It was at that point I realized how much my view of the practice of medicine had changed. This was what I wanted for myself: to get out of my computer room and back into the exam room. *I wanted to help people.*

When I got back to my office, my level of comfort in prescribing LDN was considerably increased. I decided that I needed to tell more people about LDN. I typed up a patient information page in a question-and-answer format. When I saw patients who seemed like good candidates for treatment with LDN, I told them about the treatment and gave them the information. Many patients were interested.

Currently, I have over one hundred patients taking LDN. The results I've seen far exceed anything that could be attributed to a placebo effect. Because I have a general internal medicine practice, I see a wide variety of illnesses, many of them chronic. This has given me the opportunity to try out LDN in many clinical situations and monitor the response.

I have used LDN for autoimmune joint diseases, including rheumatoid arthritis, psoriatic arthritis, lupus, and ankylosing spondylitis. I have used it for inflammatory bowel disease, celiac disease, and irritable bowel syndrome. I have also used it for chronic-pain syndromes such as fibromyalgia, neuropathic pain, chronic regional pain syndrome, and osteoarthritis. Other disorders such as fatigue, asthma, allergies, and dermatitis have also responded. These illnesses may all look different on the surface, but the underlying problems are the same. Most chronic diseases have a component of inflammation and immune system dysfunction. LDN works at the root of the problem, addressing the core issues, resulting in improvement in the clinical syndrome.

I have one patient with stage one prostate cancer who prior to seeing me was being treated with expectant management alone (also known as watchful waiting). We started LDN and watched his PSA (prostate cancer tumor marker) drop by over 20% in two months. Six months later it had dropped again, and we are continuing to monitor it.

I have kept careful records and maintain a spreadsheet on my computer of all my patients taking LDN, detailing their diagnoses and progress. As a very conservative figure, at least 70% of the patients who have tried LDN have had a clinical response. If you take out the patients who stopped early because of side effects, the number increases to over 80%. Of the patients who have had a clinical response, the percentage who rate their response as much improved (which would be a level 5 on a scale of 1 to 5) is around 30%.

Not everyone has had a dramatic response, but there are many who have. Some of my patients became symptom-free within just a few months of treatment. Some of my chronic-pain patients were pain-free within the first month. It has been an amazing thing to witness, and every day I am thankful to have the opportunity to watch the responses as they happen. I am grateful to my original patient who first introduced me to LDN. I am grateful to all the pioneer physicians who have gone before me, and I am deeply humbled to be able to tell my story in their company.

A lot has changed in my life since I got that first stethoscope. A lot has changed since my days of wanting to walk away from medicine. My sense of hope has been renewed, and I love being a doctor again. My sincere desire is for other doctors to also have their lives and practices renewed. I want more patients to know about LDN and have the opportunity to try it if they might benefit. I want to help spread the word, and thanks to Linda Elsegood and the LDN Research Trust, this book is an important step in that direction.

In the following pages, many different experts tell their stories about how low dose naltrexone has made a difference in their areas of expertise. Information is presented about LDN's development, pharmacology, clinical trials, efficacy in the treatment of various disorders, and current areas of ongoing study. Our hope is to educate clinicians and give them the information and tools they need to feel comfortable incorporating treatment with LDN into their practices. We are also expecting that a number of patients will be interested in this information as well, and that the book can open a door of communication between patients and their clinicians in a positive way, as we work together toward our common goal of healing.

JILL COTTEL, MD
MEDICAL DIRECTOR, POWAY INTEGRATIVE
MEDICINE CENTER, POWAY, CA

ONE

The History and Pharmacology of LDN

J. STEPHEN DICKSON,
BSC (HONS), MRPHARMS

Naltrexone belongs to a class of drugs called opiate antagonists, a relatively new class of medicines that were first formally theorized in the 1940s. Antagonists, including opiate antagonists, block the physiological activity of other drugs, as well as naturally occurring hormones, catecholamines, peptides, and neurotransmitters.

Among the first classes of antagonists to be developed were the beta-blockers, discovered by Sir James W. Black in 1964. Beta-blockers, such as propranolol, are adrenergic blocking drugs, used to control the "fight or flight" response in human beings. The discovery of propranolol is widely heralded as the most important contribution to pharmacology in the twentieth century.[1]

Being able to modify endogenous biological mechanisms in a clinically relevant way was so important to medicine that in 1988 the decision was made to award Sir Black with the Nobel Prize in Medicine, not only for his development of antagonists but for his follow-up work, which showed how blocking receptor sites (in this case adrenergic receptors) could be used for the management of debilitating conditions, including high blood pressure, angina pectoris, and heart failure. To this day, beta-blockers are the mainstay of treatment for patients with cardiac problems, preventing millions of deaths worldwide since their development, making them one of the most successful classes of drugs ever produced.[2] The scientific excitement generated by the potential of receptors to treat disease led researchers to look closely at how opiate painkillers actually worked in relation to opioid receptors in the body.

Painkillers based on the opium poppy (*Papaver somniferum*) have existed for millennia, as evidenced in literature by Homer's *Odyssey*, written nearly three thousand years ago: "Presently she cast a drug into the wine of which they drank to lull all pain and anger and bring forgetfulness of every sorrow."[3] Although Theophrastus in 300 BC, and Diskourides in AD 60, both argued that the wine in question was actually an extract of the henbane plant, which contains several active tropane alkaloids (notably scopolamine, hyoscine, and atropine, the latter of which will be discussed later in this chapter), this has been refuted in modern times, with pharmacologists Schmiedeberg (1918) and Lewin (1931) making a convincing case that Helena's drink in the *Odyssey* was made from the extract of the opium poppy.[4]

Archaeologists have also uncovered many references to painkillers made from the opium poppy. Six-thousand-year-old Sumerian texts and two-thousand-year-old Egyptian hieroglyphs contain similar symbols referring to *gil*, which, when translated into modern language, stands for *joy* and is derived from *hul gil*, whose pictograph is unmistakably an opium poppy.[5]

Many references throughout history support the common use of opiates for a variety of ailments. The Ebers Papyrus, dated approximately 1500 BC, recommends a particular remedy to "prevent excessive crying of children" and includes instructions for how to make it: "Spenn, the grains of the spenn [poppy]-plant, with excretions of flies found on the wall, strained to a pulp, passed through a sieve and administered on four successive days. The crying will stop at once."[6]

The Greco-Roman fascination with opium is clear in many historical records. In ancient Greece, Hippocrates (460 BC) made many medicinal treatments from herbs, including the opium poppy seed.[7] Opium abuse is also widespread in every time period from which records exist. Notably, Roman Emperor Marcus Aurelius displayed many of the symptoms and side effects of opium addiction.[8] The decline of the Roman Empire, which began in about AD 500, took with it many trade routes, and widespread knowledge of the opium poppy appears to have retreated back to the Arab world for the next few hundred years.

The opium poppy has been cultivated in the Arab world continuously since ancient times. Records of cultivation most often point to the country now known as Iraq, previously Sumeria, with good evidence of post–Roman

Empire trade networks for opium poppies and their extracts beginning to India and China in AD 800 and further into what is now Europe by AD 1500.[9] The spread of opium as a recreational drug, which was most often smoked, is frequently attributed to this exponential growth and advance of Arabian influence from AD 500 to AD 1000. With the foundation and rise of Islam, Arab peoples commonly used both opium and hashish recreationally due to the prohibition of alcohol in the Koran.[10] Manuscripts referring to widespread common usage of opium, both medicinal and recreational, start to appear more regularly in the historical record from AD 1500 onward.[11] Paracelsus, a Swiss doctor often heralded as the father of modern medicine, first standardized an alcoholic extract of the opium poppy, known as laudanum, in 1527.[12] This standardized laudanum has been in use right up to the modern era, with the first branded laudanum making an appearance in England in as early as 1680.[13]

It is notable, and very important to the development of naltrexone, that the use of opium extracts was commonly known to result in addiction as well as death by overdose. Surgeons routinely used opiate extracts to dull pain or perform surgery, but due to the unpredictable nature of the strength of the opiates in medicines, death from overdose during surgery occurred frequently. The use of *spongia somnifera* (a sponge soaked in opium used locally during surgery, considered to be a safer alternative to large oral doses of opium) was commonplace until modern times, but was often ineffective due to lack of absorption,[14] or too effective, causing complications.[15]

It was not until the Georgian Era (1740–1830) that the modern science of chemistry was sufficiently advanced to allow fractional distillation, as well as extraction and identification, of active components. German pharmacist Friedrich Sertürner first isolated opium's active component in an extract called papaverine in 1806 and named it morphine, after the Greek god Morpheus, the god of dreams.[16] Morphine belongs to a class of substances known as alkaloids. The term *alkaloid* was first used in 1819 by Swiss botanist Carl Meissner when he referred to a plant known as *al-qali*.[17] Sodium carbonate, first extracted from this plant, was known as *al-kali* in Arabic. The term has come to refer to a chemical's pH and, unsurprisingly, alkaloids are slightly alkaline.

The discovery of a natural, active component that could be extracted and purified generated much scientific excitement. But at this stage of history, the science of receptors was nonexistent, and an understanding of how the drug worked was less important to the scientists of the day than producing stronger, more powerful versions with fewer side effects.

Morphine continued to be extracted and widely used throughout the first part of the nineteenth century. Additionally, the use of morphine as an adjunct to chloroform for anesthesia started to become widespread in the 1850s after being popularized by French physiologist Claude Bernard.[18] Bernard's experiments on animals demonstrated empirically that less chloroform was needed to keep an animal anesthetized when it was premedicated with morphine.[19]

However, over the next fifty years it became increasingly apparent to doctors that morphine had several drawbacks, including breathing suppression, constipation, addiction, and even death by overdose. As morphine's problems became more widely known and understood, an intense search began to find safer alternatives.

English scientist Charles Romley Alder Wright first synthesized di-acetyl-morphine in 1874 by chemically adding two acetyl groups to the morphine molecule, now commonly known as diamorphine or, when abused, heroin.[20] Over the next few decades many such chemical analogues of the original morphine were made, each one heralded as the "new morphine" without the side effects or drawbacks. None of these new compounds were found to be free of side effects, and it is now known that the beneficial effects of morphine analogues are directly tied to the side effects through the same receptors.

Research continued, but during World War I (1914–1918) many developed countries found it difficult to access morphine due to disrupted trade. The lessened availability of morphine intensified the scientific search for a way to synthesize the drug. Throughout World War II, difficulties obtaining morphine during the previous war were acutely remembered, but by this time another chemical took the spotlight: atropine.

Atropine is extracted from the belladonna plant (*Atropa belladonna*), a perennial plant native to parts of Europe and western Asia. Historically, it was used in medieval times to increase the size of women's pupils, which led to its name (*bella*: beautiful, *donna*: woman), but it would later prove to have much more important uses. At the time of the war effort, atropine was the only anti-cholinergic agent available to medics to counteract an attack with nerve gas. Since an inability to source sufficient atropine would significantly disadvantage any army, huge resources were applied to find an alternative to plant-derived atropine on both sides of the war.

It was through this intense scientific effort that a German scientist, Dr. Otto Eisleb, first synthesized a molecule that he called meperidine, in 1939. Meperidine failed to successfully replace atropine, but was soon recognized by Dr. Otto Schumann (who was working for a German chemical company, IG Farben) as a powerful analgesic, similar in action to morphine.[21] Meperidine is still used today during childbirth, and is commonly known as pethidine. Pethidine represented the first opiate drug with a chemical structure completely divergent from that of morphine (see figure 1.1).

The door to chemical synthesis of new drug compounds was now well and truly open, with scientific laboratories working around the clock synthesizing new compounds. The next most widely known nonmorphine opiate to be discovered was 1,1-diphenyl-1 (dimethylaminoisopropyl) butanone-2, now commonly known as methadone, synthesized just a few short years later between 1940 and 1946.[22]

Working in the research laboratories of Merck & Co., two scientists, Weijlard and Erikson,[23] synthesized another compound, which puzzled everyone. In certain circumstances, this compound seemed to exert the opposite effect of morphine, reversing the latter's negative effects. They called this compound nalorphine (chemical name N-allylnormorphine). Weijlard and Erikson discovered that this compound actually had mixed effects: It had a slight analgesic action in animals, a bit like morphine, but

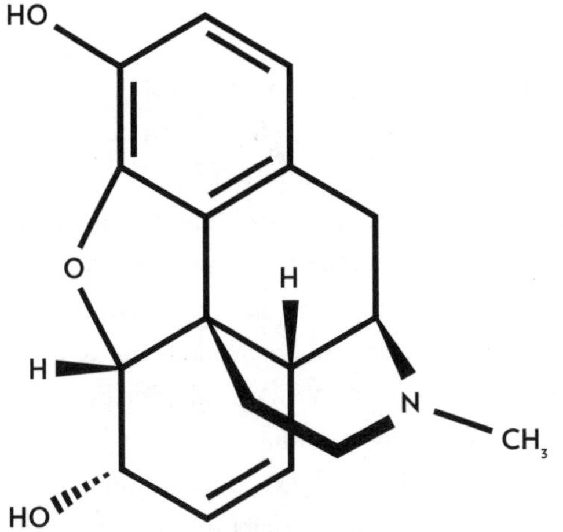

FIGURE 1.1. Structure of morphine.

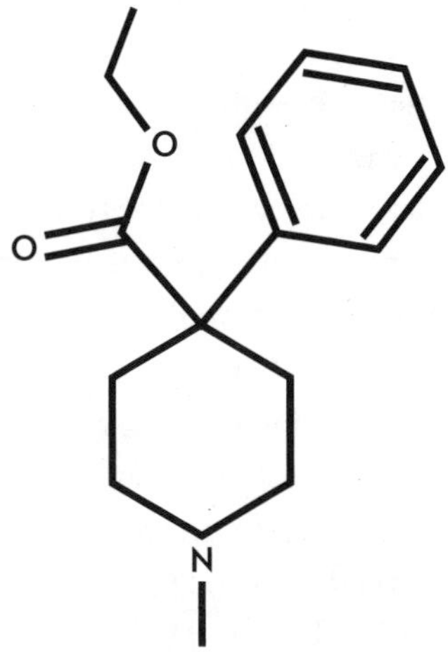

FIGURE 1.2. Structure of pethedine.

when given to an animal pretreated with an overdose of morphine, the effects of the morphine (such as breathing suppression) were reversed. This discovery presented a bit of a conundrum, as medical science did not yet understand the concept of receptors.

However, unhindered by the confusing effects of this compound, and recognizing that a drug that completely blocks the negative effects of morphine would be very useful, many laboratories and companies continued to synthesize different molecules. The first patent for a pure morphine-blocking drug was recorded in Great Britain in 1963,[24] and in the United States in 1966.[25] The discovered compound was naloxone.

Naloxone was a panacea for opiate overdose. Upon intravenous injection, it appeared to immediately block all effects of morphine. Fifty years later, naloxone is still on the World Health Organization's international list of essential medicines.[26]

More importantly to the background of low dose naltrexone (LDN), naloxone's discovery led to other researchers discovering an analog in 1967, which could be taken orally, named "Endo 1639A".[27] Endo 1639A is now commonly known as naltrexone.

Historical Use of Naltrexone

Addiction to opiate drugs has long been a societal problem. People become addicted to opiate medications for a number of reasons: They numb physical and psychological pain; with long-term use, they cause biological changes that result in side effects upon withdrawal; and they create pharmacological tolerance, requiring ever-larger doses to produce a similar effect.

It is important to understand some of the underlying biological mechanisms that are involved in the action of opiates in order to understand the importance of the naltrexone molecule. Opiate medications, as well as opiate-acting medications that have the same effect but a different structure (such as pethidine, described above), mimic natural neuropeptides. These natural neuropeptides are called endorphins, and specifically in the case of opiate analgesic actions, beta-endorphins. They are synthesized in the brain in the anterior pituitary gland and are released in reaction to a variety of stimuli.

The precursor protein to most endorphins is POMC (pro-opiomelano-cortin). In normal physiological function, the hypothalamus secretes CRH (corcitrophin-releasing hormone) in response to stress on the physiological system. This in turn stimulates the pituitary to make POMC, which, as a large complex molecule, can be enzymatically broken up into neuropeptides such as the endorphins. A negative feedback loop then occurs, which suppresses the release of CRH when the by-products of POMC breakdown reach a certain level. Almost every physiological system in the body contains the necessary enzymes to break down POMC to the component neuropeptides.

When discussing how endorphins work, it is perhaps simplest to focus on their painkilling (analgesic) properties. These are generally well understood and have a sound scientific literature. They may have a much more complex biological role, which is less understood, but this will be discussed later.

There are two main areas of action for analgesia where natural endogenous neuropeptides, such as beta-endorphins, exert a painkilling effect: first, the peripheral nervous system (PNS) and second, the central nervous system (CNS).

The PNS can be thought of metaphorically as the wires connecting every part of the human body between sensors and the brain. These wires are connected together via junctions. However, unlike in an electrical system—where the wires touch each other—nerve junctions speak to each other via the release of chemicals. These chemicals are called neurotransmitters. A nerve can be described as starting with a postsynaptic terminal, which receives messages from the previous nerve, and ending with a presynaptic terminal, to communicate with the next nerve. The nerves that transmit the sensation of pain do so by releasing a neurotransmitter called "Substance P." In the PNS, opiates bind mainly to the presynaptic terminal and prevent the release of Substance P by a cascade reaction. If Substance P cannot be released into the nerve junction, the pain signal cannot be transmitted.

Diagrammatically, this is difficult to represent in a simple manner. However, returning to simplified university lecture notes, the reaction can be represented as shown in figure 1.3.

In figure 1.3 we see how communication of the pain signal is interrupted by the naturally occurring endorphins, which act on opiate receptors to suppress pain in a similar way to opiate drugs. In this way, a pain signal coming from the peripheral sensing systems can be prevented from being as strong when it makes it back to the brain, or even from making it to the brain at all.

This system is far more complex than is represented here; there are a range of neurotransmitters called tachykinins that act in similar ways to Substance P, along with several different types of opiate receptor, each of which has a slightly different action and all of which are involved in the chemical cascade that fully transmits pain throughout the different nerve fibers in the PNS. However, a subclass of opiate receptors called "mu" receptors is ubiquitous through the PNS and is the main target for opiate analgesics.

In the CNS, specifically the brain, opiate receptors are very well distributed and are involved in a multitude of different neurochemical actions. Unlike the PNS, opiate receptors centrally act to inhibit pain by modifying the release of the potent neurotransmitter dopamine.

Dopamine is commonly known as the body's natural "happy chemical" and is primarily controlled by the release of another neurotransmitter called GABA (gamma-aminobutyric acid). When opiates bind to the mu-opioid receptor, they cause a reduction in the release of GABA, which in turn reduces the inhibitory effect that GABA activation has on the presynaptic nerve release of dopamine.

In layman's terms, activating a mu-opioid receptor centrally disrupts the normal controls on baseline release of dopamine, meaning that far

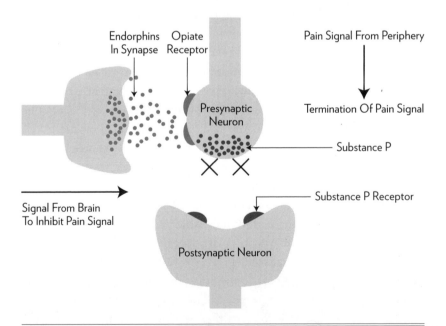

FIGURE 1.3. Communication of pain signal interrupted by endorphins.

more dopamine is released than normal. This has an analgesic effect by suppressing the conduction of pain messages and the response to pain caused by the euphoric effect of excess dopamine. The excess dopamine is largely responsible for the "high" desired by people who abuse opiates, but belongs entirely to a natural system that exists to maintain homeostasis and is activated by naturally occurring endorphins as discussed earlier.

A diagram showing this process at work will help to make this process clearer.

In figure 1.4, normal homoeostasis is depicted on the left. On the right, heroin (diamorphine), breaks down to morphine and then attaches to a mu-opioid receptor, inhibiting GABA release, and increasing dopamine release. The mu-opioid receptors on these nerves are activated by biological endorphins.

Receptors are one of the most important discoveries in modern medicine. Although theorized widely in the 1960s, the first opiate receptor was discovered in the early 1970s when the technology of radioisotope labeling became available.[28] Interestingly, the scientists who are widely referred to as

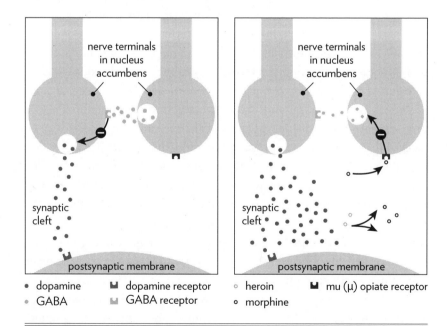

FIGURE 1.4. *Left*, normal function of GABA and mu-opioid receptors. *Right*, effect of heroin on GABA and mu-opioid receptors.

the first to describe and identify an opiate receptor did so using naloxone, which, as discussed earlier, led directly to the development of naltrexone.

It has since been discovered that many receptors are similar in nature, and in fact, opiate receptors belong to a family called G-protein-coupled receptors, which are all generally inhibitory when activated. Structurally, opioid receptors are similar to somatostatin receptors and another class of receptor, which will be discussed later, called toll-like receptors (TLR), that are involved in inflammatory processes.[29]

Returning to the opioid receptors, scientists quickly discovered that many different chemicals could bind to them. Although some chemicals could bind to the receptors and be observed attaching to the receptor via radiological study, they did not all have the same effect. In fact, a huge range of activity was seen, ranging from extreme activation of the receptor, to slight activation, and right up to blocking anything else from attaching to the receptor. In pharmacology, chemicals that produce these effects are referred to, respectively, as agonists, partial agonists, and antagonists.

Classically, receptors are thought of as locks. Imagine a standard door lock where different keys can fit into the same keyhole. Agonists are keys that fit the lock and open the door fully (extreme activation of the receptor); partial agonists fit the lock but only partially open the door (slight activation); and antagonists fit the lock, but cannot open the door, actively preventing any other keys from trying to open the door (blocking).

Figure 1.5 shows that although the lock (receptor) and key (ligand) analogy is easy to understand, the actual structure of a receptor site is in three dimensions, and different parts of the receptor can be activated or blocked depending on the physical structure of the ligand interacting with it. Endogenous endorphins, such as the beta-endorphins discussed earlier, are agonists; these are mimicked by opiate drugs such as morphine and diamorphine. Naltrexone and naloxone are antagonists: keys that fit the same door, but stop the receptor from being activated by an agonist. It has since been discovered that these receptors are fluid and can become more or less sensitive to agonists and can increase and decrease in active number depending on circumstances.

Based on this knowledge, naltrexone was first licensed as a treatment for addiction to opiates in 1984.[30] Scientists understood that blocking opioid receptors would prevent an addicted patient from being able to obtain the euphoria achieved by taking drugs such as heroin. As such, naltrexone was

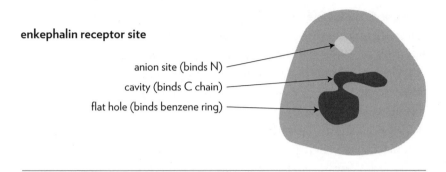

FIGURE 1.5. Enkephalin receptor site. Adapted from Fred Senese; "Anandamide." General Chemistry Online! Last revised Feb. 15, 2015. http://antoine.frostburg.edu/chem/senese/101/features/anandamide.shtml.

highly effective; when a patient addicted to high doses of opiates was given naltrexone, all the effects of the opiates were immediately blocked for a number of hours. However, this efficacy proved to be highly dangerous, resulting in large numbers of deaths of patients who were tolerant to opiates and thus were unwittingly pushed into immediate opiate withdrawal.

The problem with attempting to treat addiction to opiates with an antagonist is that as someone becomes a regular user of opiates, the reactivity of the receptors to opiates (natural endorphins included) is greatly reduced, and the physical number of receptors also decreases. This is a natural biological phenomenon caused by physiology always attempting to return to a baseline state (homeostasis). In pharmacology, this effect is referred to in terms such as *desensitization* and *down-regulation*.

This is a reversible reaction, and naltrexone was used widely in the 1980s and 1990s for assistance with abstinence from opiates, but only once a patient had been gradually titrated down from their regular dose and a level homeostasis had returned. Naltrexone was given in tablet form, orally, in daily doses ranging from 50 milligrams (mg) to 300 mg. The opiate receptor blockade was strong and predictable; should the patient take any opiates while on naltrexone, there was no euphoric effect.

Still, there were several problems that led to naltrexone not becoming the mainstay for opiate addiction management. First, although the drug effectively created an opiate blockade, the patient's underlying psychological addiction to the euphoric feeling of opiates was not reduced. In fact, the cravings were often reported to be higher during naltrexone therapy.

Second, the opiate blockade in patients taking naltrexone also muted the effects of naturally occurring endorphins required to maintain a basic homeostasis. When the brain responds to pleasurable stimuli, the response is mediated by endorphins, so when full opiate blockade is achieved, it theoretically interferes with the ability of the patient to feel or experience happiness and pleasure. Opiate-addicted patients taking naltrexone often describe a "flatness," technically described as dysphoria, which is reported to lead to significant depression. The link between naltrexone and dysphoria has been researched, but results are contradictory, though dysphoria is still listed on the summary of product characteristics as a side effect. Recent research has suggested that initial symptoms of depression may improve and clinically reported side effects are related to the withdrawal from opiates, or concomitant disease.[31]

Finally, compliance with treatment was often poor due to chaotic lifestyles, or the side effects mentioned, whether real or psychosomatic; patients were often not taking the tablets every day and would therefore be able to regress into addiction. Many drug companies have tried to avoid this problem by developing a slow-release injectable pellet, a few of which are still on the market today, but the uptake has been poor due to the complexity of administration, the price of the injectable, and the overall evidence-based, international move to replacement and slow-reduction therapy with agents such as methadone.

During the period when naltrexone was being used for opiate addiction, it gained favor for treatment in another area: alcoholism. Clinicians postulated that if a patient was to take naltrexone while drinking to excess, as in the case of alcoholism, their brain could be retrained to attain no pleasure from the alcohol, by the same process as described above, blocking the effects of endorphins.

When doctors tried this in patients, they found significant success, and naltrexone has consistently gained momentum over the last twenty years as a treatment to reduce heavy drinking in alcohol-dependent patients. A review study in 2006 showed that 70% of clinical trials conducted in this area demonstrated clinically important benefit.

The basic scientific groundwork and standardization for widespread use of naltrexone for alcoholism was set out by John David Sinclair when working at the Finnish National Institute for Health and Welfare in the late 1990s. He demonstrated that a process described as "pharmacological extinction" showed that concomitant alcohol drinking when being prescribed naltrexone worked by gradually reducing the craving. Statistically, this followed an extinction curve, which was repeatable and predictable. This was named "The Sinclair Method" and is widely used throughout the world today. Sinclair's groundwork has led to a recent formal license for an analog of naltrexone, nalmefene, to be formally approved for use in patients with alcohol dependence.

Immunological Effects

Naltrexone has a long history of safe use in patients for its opiate receptor and endorphin-modifying properties. In the last decade, it has been recognized that naltrexone also has immunological effects that have been reported to be beneficial in autoimmune diseases. Furthermore, various clinicians have reported that naltrexone has also been useful in treating various types of cancer. This has led many to wonder "what is going on?" How can a medication with a well-defined and understood pharmacological effect have such a wide range of other possible indications?

Drug companies go to great lengths to modify their products before they reach licensure, to make sure the active molecule is as selective as possible for the intended target. However, despite the best efforts of drug companies, most licensed drugs on the market today are not 100% selective for their intended target.

Many biologically active chemical substances have more than one area that they will interact with in the human body. The pharmacological term for this is "dirty drug," which means that although the drug does exactly what it says it does, it also does something else. These are interpreted as "side effects," as often the secondary action is unwanted.

Over the last fifty years, the understanding of receptor structure has greatly improved as the understanding of biological "chirality" has increased dramatically. Chirality means that receptors, and other target cellular areas, are generally three dimensional structures that can be "left-handed" or "right-handed." Despite having the same cellular building blocks, they can be put together in different ways, just as our hands have the same number of bones and tendons, but are the opposite of each other.

This concept extends down to the molecular level in physiological systems, and has been discovered to be important in the production of drugs, as these too can have a "left-handed" or "right-handed" design. Chemically, this "handedness" is described as an L or R isomer.

Unsurprisingly, pharmacologists now understand that each different isomer can actually have a different effect, and the amount of drug that is bioavailable of each isomer can be dose dependent. However, most drugs, when synthesized, are present in a consistent ratio of L and R isomers in the eventual product.

Figure 1.6 serves to demonstrate that how drug molecules actually affect the human body has yet to be fully understood, and that many molecules that were previously thought to be well explained have been observed to have different effects when examined carefully for their inherent structure, or dosing regimen. As discussed earlier, drugs that alter homeostasis also have the potential for altering those inherent biological systems in different ways depending on how effective they are at modifying the natural control mechanisms.

In the case of naltrexone, the dose that seems to have an effect in autoimmune diseases is significantly lower (ten to forty times lower) than the dose used for opiate addiction or alcoholism. This is referred to as low dose naltrexone (LDN). Most commonly, LDN is taken daily in doses of between 0.5 mg and 4.5 mg.

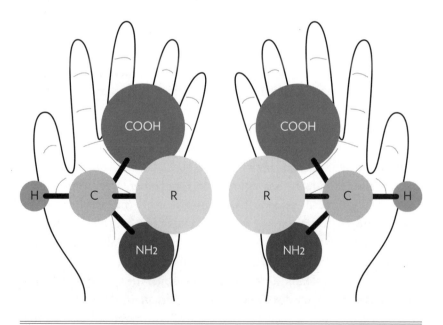

FIGURE 1.6. Demonstration of chirality. Image courtesy of NASA

LDN should not be confused with homeopathy, where an active substance is mysteriously diluted so many times that few, if any, of the original chemical molecules remain in the eventual product. Even at low doses of 0.5 mg to 4.5 mg, naltrexone still has significant bioavailability and can precipitate immediate short-term opiate withdrawal. That is to say, although the dose is a lot lower than the drug was historically licensed for, clinicians can still demonstrate some of the well-known effects of the drug at this dose. It is still biologically active at these dose ranges.

One of the first hints as to how LDN could potentially affect the immune system came from research into the effects of endorphins conducted in the early 1980s. One influential paper, published in 1985, concluded that "endorphins can be considered as immunomodulators . . . and may become a tool in the field of immunotherapy."[32] It was already known at the time that naltrexone was capable of binding to endorphin receptors, as endorphins are endogenous opiates. What was also known was that interrupting homeostasis, by blocking these receptors, could result in tricking the body to produce more endorphins to compensate.[33]

The first clinician to record immunological effects of LDN was Dr. Bernard Bihari, working in New York City in 1985. He was embroiled in the middle of the HIV/AIDS epidemic at a time when none of the modern treatments had yet been developed. Human immunodeficiency virus (HIV) is an infection that leads to destruction and weakening of the immune system; when patients become immuno-compromised, they are then said to have AIDS, the final stage of the infection, and they generally die from complications of the immune system damage. Bihari's practice tried anything and everything in this patient group to improve survival. Knowing from previously conducted research[34] that endorphins were significantly involved in the regulation of the immune system, it was an ingenious step to try treatment with LDN.

First, Dr. Bihari tested a small group of very unwell AIDS patients, whose endorphin levels were about a third of what is considered normal. This endorphin deficiency was something that his clinic felt could be treated with a small dose of naltrexone, so they began a twelve-week trial. In the placebo group, 5 out of 16 patients developed opportunistic infections, but none of the 22 in the LDN group did. These results, although on a small scale, were extremely encouraging. Bihari's clinic then proceeded to look at treating larger numbers of patients with LDN.[35]

Dr. Bihari was able to demonstrate, in a reasonably sized HIV/AIDS patient group, that taking LDN regularly largely prevented the gradual destruction of the immune system. He did this by measuring the presence in the blood of a type of immune cell called CD4. CD4 was, and remains, the standard marker for seeing how fast HIV is progressing. What was most interesting and striking in his practice was that the number of deaths in the patient group who took LDN, compared to the patient group who did not regularly take it, was vastly lower. Its success also appeared to be synergistic with the new classes of antiretroviral drugs that became available during the years of treatment, meaning that LDN improved the outcomes in his patients, regardless of whether they took the new antiretroviral drugs.[36]

Over the next few years, a plethora of research was conducted on the importance of endorphins and opiates/opiate antagonists to the regulation of the immune system. One of the most important discoveries was published in 1986 by Drs. Zagon and McLaughlin, demonstrating that opiate receptors were present inside multiple types of immune cells, and laterally that mRNA inside these cells held coding for endorphin receptors.[37]

Over the next twenty-nine years, Dr. Ian Zagon championed the basic research into endorphins and naltrexone (LDN), publishing nearly three hundred papers on the subject. The extent of the research is too overwhelming to present here; however, it has confirmed beyond doubt that the endorphin/opioid receptor system is involved in almost every biological system that regulates immune response.

The mechanism of action of LDN, as proposed by these studies, can be summarized as follows:

1. Many outward diseases are expressions of a malfunctioning immune system.
2. The immune system is regulated by endorphins, which have a primary action on opiate receptors.
3. Blocking opiate receptors briefly using naltrexone causes an up-regulation in the production of endorphins, which can act in an immunomodulatory way to correct immune system malfunction.
4. Furthermore, cell growth (proliferation) is also mediated by a subtype of endorphins; cell proliferation can be suppressed by endorphins, and this is applicable to some forms of cancer.[38]

This is a gross simplification of thirty years of detailed work, of course, and to fully understand the concepts within the published papers would take a degree in immunology and a lot of time. However, the experimental models for multiple sclerosis; wound healing; pancreatic, colon, brain, head/neck, liver, breast, and ovarian cancers; ocular surface disease; Crohn's disease; and many other pathways, have been shown to be responsive to endorphins in vitro. The wide range of diseases that appear to be responsive to modification of the endorphin system is staggering, none more so than terminal cancers and debilitating autoimmune diseases like multiple sclerosis.

Over the last twenty-five years, clinical use of LDN has been increasing. However, many researchers currently think that endorphins are not the whole picture. Scientists have long known that naltrexone binds to more than just the opiate receptors; there is also a significant attachment to a group of receptors called toll-like receptors (TLRs).

Toll-like receptors were first demonstrated in 1985 by Christiane Nüsslein-Volhard.[39] They are an essential part of the innate immune system, providing a first line of defense against microbial invasion, and are present on cells such as white blood cells (macrophages), dendritic cells, neutrophils, B lymphocytes, mast cells, and monocytes, as well as directly on cells of various human organs, such as the kidney and intestines.

When a foreign body invades, such as bacteria, different subclasses of TLR receptors (TLR-1 to TLR-10 in humans) respond to different parts of the invading organism, including surface proteins, by-products from the cellular metabolism of the bacteria/virus, physical structures on the surface or inside of the bacterial cell, DNA, RNA, and even the specific sugars that are unique to certain bacteria. This is not an exhaustive list, as research continues to this day. For example, a class of TLR receptor (TLR-10) is known to exist, but the substrate is not presently known.

The role of these receptors appears to be to recognize an intruder—they have a structure complimentary to doing so—and then to start an intercellular signaling pathway that triggers an appropriate immune response.

In general, activation of a TLR leads to the production of pro-inflammatory cytokines (a loose class of small proteins), which then mobilize the innate immune system to, for example, send white blood cells to the affected area to engulf the intruder—or in the case of a virus, instruct the infected cell to die. Interestingly, the activation of many types of TLRs has been demon-strated to also produce a highly potent molecule called NF-kB (pronounced enn-eff-kappa-bee) as part of the signaling mechanism.[40] NF-kB is currently undergoing intense research and has been shown to be a potent target for the treatment of autoimmune diseases and cancers.[41] NF-kB has even been linked to the expression of cancer oncogenes, which turn off the natural cell-death mechanism, leading to the uncontrolled growth of the cancer.[42]

As with all biological systems, TLRs appear to have more than one way of being activated. As mentioned previously, naltrexone is a potent antag-onist of the TLR receptor pathway.[43] This pathway has been shown to be clinically relevant in vivo, by studies showing that naltrexone can inhibit TLR-4 and reverse symptoms of neuropathic pain.[44]

A recent paper specifically discussing neuropathic pain was one of the first to demonstrate that the effect of naltrexone is chiral. Returning to an earlier discussion, where left- and right-handed molecules can have different bind-ing sites, a study by Hutchinson and colleagues in 2008 effectively demon-strated that opiate-binding receptors are antagonized by *levo*-naltrexone, whereas the TLR-4 receptor is antagonized by *dextro*-naltrexone.[45]

It is entirely possible, and in fact likely, that the reason naltrexone seems to have such a wide range of activity in different physiological systems is because it behaves as two different drugs, depending on struc-ture of the isomer.

Clinicians and scientists postulate that in some autoimmune diseases, such as lupus, rheumatoid arthritis, and multiple sclerosis, natural mamma-lian cell by-products may inappropriately activate TLR receptors, directly leading to the inappropriate inflammation.[46] In addition, imiquimod, a drug that has recently reached clinical use for treating skin cancer, has been shown to activate, rather than antagonize, TLR-7, causing so much inflammation in the area that it is very effective at killing basal cell cancer of the skin.[47]

To summarize the data so far:

- Naltrexone, when produced for human consumption, consists of a 50:50 mixture of levo- and dextro-isomers.
- Levo-naltrexone is an antagonist for the opiate/endorphin receptors, and is credited with:
  – Up-regulation of endorphin release;
  – Immunomodulation; and

TABLE 1.1. Forms and Dosages of LDN

Dosage Form	Dosage Range	Usage
4.5 mg capsules	Commonly 1, but up to 4 capsules taken morning or night, or morning and night.	Autoimmune diseases, cancer, chronic fatigue syndrome.
3 mg capsules	Commonly 1, but up to 4 capsules taken morning or night, or morning and night.	Autoimmune diseases, cancer, chronic fatigue syndrome.
Liquid 1 mg/1 ml	0.5 mg–20 mg taken orally. Morning and/or night.	Usually used for initiation, to titrate patient up to 3 mg or 4.5 mg. Often patient cannot tolerate an exact capsules dose and will remain on liquid indefinitely. Used more commonly with chronic fatigue syndrome (CFS) and Hashimoto's disease, as patients often respond to lower doses.
Sublingual drops 10 mg/ml	0.5 mg–20 mg taken under tongue. Usually once daily.	Used to avoid some first-pass metabolism, where gastrointestinal side effects have been severe, or no effect has been visible with standard dosing.
Cream 0.5 mg–10 mg/ml	Dose range varies between 0.5 mg and 4.5 mg daily.	Used originally for autistic children. Commonly used in patients who cannot tolerate oral dosage forms. Bioavailability of this formulation is highly doubtful. Topically, in sterile form, it may be useful to promote wound healing.*

* I. S. Zagon et al., "Naltrexone Accelerates Healing without Compromise of Adhesion Complexes in Normal and Diabetic Corneal Epithelium," *Brain Research Bulletin* 72, no. 1 (April 2007): 18–24.

      – Reductions in cell proliferation via endorphins.
- Dextro-naltrexone is an antagonist for at least one, if not more, TLRs, and is reported to:
  - Antagonize TLR, suppressing cytokine modulated immune system; and
  - Antagonize TLR-mediated production of NF-kB, reducing inflammation, and potentially down-regulating oncogenes.

In this way, it is easy to see how the large number of actions attributed to LDN could be feasible. What is currently lacking is sufficient in vivo,

TABLE 1.2. Potential Side Effects of LDN

Side Effects	Length of Duration
Nightmares, insomnia, vivid dreams	During initial phase and can be persistent in some patients.
Stomach cramps/diarrhea	Transitory, up to 2 weeks usually.
Headache	During initial phase only.
Hyperthyroidism	Can come on very quickly if concurrent with Hashimoto's disease.
Shivers, chills, flu-like symptoms	Most common in myalgic encephalomyelitis (ME) and chronic fatigue syndrome (CFS) patients.
Agitation or dizziness, extrapyramidal symptoms	Infrequent.
Constipation and/or diarrhea	Infrequent. More common in irritable bowel syndrome (IBS)/inflammatory bowel disease (IBD)/ulcerative colitis and Crohn's disease.
Elevated liver enzymes	Very infrequent. Usually when patient has late-stage liver failure.
Reductions in renal function	Extremely rare.

Source: "Naltrexone Hydrochloride 50 mg Film-Coated Tablets," medicines.org.uk, last updated March 5, 2014, https://www.medicines.org.uk/emc/medicine/25878.

double-blind clinical studies, showing that the effects proven in a petri dish and test tube scale up reliably to actions on humans.

Dosage and Route of Administration

LDN is administered in many different forms and dosages. These are listed in table 1.1 in approximate order of popularity.

Low dose naltrexone is commonly started once daily, at 0.5 to 1.5 mg. This is to allow the clinician to evaluate how the patient will respond. Side effects, as reported by patients, can often be prevented by the patient starting at a low dosage and increasing by 1 mg per week until reaching 4.5 mg. In the

Action Required

Switch to taking LDN in the morning.

None. Potentially take a fiber supplement daily. Probably caused by TLR receptor in intestine, or antagonism of delta-opiate receptors altering bowel contractions.

Self-limiting and goes away after a few days in most people.

Never increase dose by more than 0.5 mg weekly in Hashimoto's disease and watch for hyperthyroid symptoms, reducing thyroid replacement therapy as required.

If persists longer than 24 hours, half the current dose of LDN and stay on half until symptoms improve. Continue with titration upward after symptoms resolve. Repeat if it happens again.

Parkinson's disease patients may experience a surge in dopamine levels due to endorphin release. Modification of dopamine-replacement therapy and monitoring required.
If patient does not have Parkinson's disease and exhibits extrapyramidal symptoms, LDN is then contraindicated.

Treat symptomatically.

Halve dose and monitor. Usually transitory.
Initial monitoring of liver enzymes rarely necessary, but up to individual clinician and caution should be exercised in patients with advanced liver disease.

Monitor carefully in chronic kidney disease (CKD) stage 3 or later (moderate to severe failure). Not a specific contraindication to treatment.

Note: Readers should note that this is not an exhaustive list; it is recommended that readers reference the summary of product characteristics for naltrexone for a full list of possible side effects.

past, scientists assumed that because the majority of LDN's assumed effects involved endorphins, it would be beneficial to take LDN at night. This belief has gradually fallen out of favor over the last five years, as clinical experience shows that the incidence of side effects is higher when LDN is taken at night, but clinical response is just as good when taken in the morning. Generally, clinicians in the United Kingdom recommend starting LDN in the morning.

Some patients, especially Crohn's disease patients, have tried taking LDN twice daily. Many have reported benefit, but this may be specific to this patient subset, due to an abundance of TLR receptors being expressed inside the small and large intestine.

Side Effects

Side effects are largely restricted to the starting phase. These are listed in table 1.2 in approximate order of how often they happen.

Combined Protocols

In addition to side effects and combined protocols, it is worth considering the safety of concomitant administration of LDN with other medications. Historically, a large amount of anecdotal evidence points toward avoiding corticosteroids while taking LDN. This has been largely refuted by recent clinical experience, where most clinicians will initiate LDN if the patient is on 20 mg or lower daily prednisolone equivalent. Furthermore, combination therapy of LDN with certain opiate-based painkillers is possible, but requires careful consideration and discussion among the health care team before initiating therapy, as LDN can stop opiate painkillers from working entirely for a short period of time and has been known to cause immediate withdrawal symptoms, even hospitalization, when started incorrectly.

Conclusion

Naltrexone has a long history of amelioration and treatment of human disease. Widespread research continues internationally into the relatively new use of LDN for immune, autoimmune, and neoplastic diseases, with sporadic use for a variety of seemingly unrelated conditions. There is significant rationale for a clinician to consider the use of LDN as an adjunct to standard therapy, where standard therapies are unsuccessful. Several clinical trials are either under design or under way as of 2016, and it is highly likely that a licensed form of LDN will be available within five years. Until

TABLE 1.3. Combined Protocols

Protocol	Disease specific	Author, popularized by or used by
LDN plus 300 mg alpha-lipoic acid (ALA-N) twice daily.	Pancreatic cancer. Hepatic cancer. Other nonspecific cancers.	Dr. Burt Berkson.[*]
LDN plus vitamin D up to 10,000 international units (IU) daily.	Autoimmune diseases. Specifically multiple sclerosis.	Various—based upon autoimmune research.[†]
LDN plus omega-3 2–4 g DHA daily	All diseases LDN is used for.	Multiple clinicians. Popularized by Dr. Thomas Gilhooly from 2000 onward. Omega-3 research.[‡]
LDN plus cannabinoids for cancer. LDN for 3 weeks, then cannabinoids for 1 week is most common therapy regimen.	Cancer therapy. Breast, lung, pancreatic, glioblastoma, and melanoma most common.	In vitro research, some of which is continuing, has shown potential synergism between cannabinoids and LDN for treating cancer.[§] Treatment break from LDN seems important in some prepublished data.

[*] B. M. Berkson, "Revisiting the ALA/N (Alpha-Lipoic Acid/Low-Dose Naltrexone) Protocol for People with Metastatic and Nonmetastatic Pancreatic Cancer: A Report of 3 New Cases," *Integrative Cancer Therapies* 8, no. 4 (December 2009): 416–422.

[†] M. F. Holick, "Sunlight and Vitamin D for Bone Health and Prevention of Autoimmune Diseases, Cancers, and Cardiovascular Diseases," *The American Journal of Clinical Nutrition* 80, no. 6 (December 2004): 1678S–1688S.

[‡] D. Swanson et al., "Omega-3 Fatty Acids EPA and DHA: Health Benefits Throughout Life," *Advances in Nutrition* 3, no. 1 (January 2012): 1–7.

[§] Ibid.

then, patients and clinicians should make an informed decision on what is most appropriate for them by looking at the currently available evidence, both published and anecdotal, before considering treatment.

Notes

Naltrexone in both standard and low dose forms is often created illegally, manufactured to substandard quality, and sold on the Internet. No reputable pharmacy will sell naltrexone without a prescription. Any patient trying to source a prescriber or supplier for LDN should refer to reputable sources. The only charity in the United Kingdom that promotes research into LDN, and has extensive links to international resources, prescribers, and suppliers, is the LDN Research Trust.

TWO

Multiple Sclerosis and Lupus

Deanna Windham, DO

W hen patients of all autoimmune diseases are combined, the number of people whose bodies are under attack from their own immune system has reached epidemic proportions. According to the American Autoimmune Related Disorders Association (AARDA), fifty million Americans have an autoimmune disease, making it the leading cause of death in females below the age of 64, and that number is on the rise. Cancer and heart disease affect nine million and twenty-three million people respectively, but research into these areas is much better funded, partially because autoimmune diseases are so complicated and include so many different disease processes. In this extended chapter I will focus on two of the most common autoimmune diseases, multiple sclerosis and lupus. But most autoimmune diseases have more similarities than differences when comparing the factors that will be discussed here, and I hope that this information will be of benefit to anyone with an autoimmune disease.

Multiple Sclerosis

Multiple sclerosis (MS) is the most common autoimmune neurodegenerative disease, with nearly 2.5 million people worldwide and 1 million people in the United States being affected, by conservative estimates, and 80% of them women. The course of disease is highly variant, but the norm is a progressive, painful, and usually debilitating neurodegenerative disorder.

The core characteristic of the disease is the destruction of the myelin sheath surrounding the nerves. The myelin sheath acts like the insulation on an electrical wire, allowing the nerve to conduct information quickly from one area to another. The myelin also provides nutrition and protection to the nerve. The destruction of this sheath and the corresponding nerve causes a disruption in the neuronal messaging both within the brain and between the brain and the body.

There are several pathological processes at work in MS:

1. *Inflammation* can potentially reduce transmission of information between neurons in at least three ways: The soluble factors released by inflammatory cells potentially stop the normal neurotransmission of intact neurons, these factors lead to or enhance the loss of myelin, or these factors may cause the axon to break down completely. The release of inflammatory cytokines (cytokines are a chemical language that cells use to communicate) is central to the process of autoreactivity and overactivation of the immune system.

2. MS is a primary *demyelinating* disease. Research has identified four types of MS when evaluated for primary pathology.[1]

   - Types I and II appear to be primarily instigated by an autoimmune attack against the myelin and oligodendrocytes (the cells that make the myelin). Some research has even shown that MS does not progress without autoreactive (self-reactive) T cells. This occurs due to a leaky blood brain barrier (BBB) through which T cells gain entry into the central nervous system (CNS) and, once there, "see" the cells in the brain for the first time and identify them as foreign. This aberrant process may also be activated by a virus or other pathogen via mimicry.

   - Types III and IV appear to start not with autoimmunity but with damage to or failure of the oligodendrocytes themselves. Oligodendrocytes are the cells that make the myelin sheath surrounding the nerve axon. Through a complex interaction with many cells and pathological processes, this culminates in a massive microglial cell activation creating worsening plaques in the CNS, brain atrophy, and neurodegenerative decay.

3. There is another aspect of MS that is *vascular*,[2] leading to BBB damage. The BBB, when damaged, allows normally excluded products in the blood stream to pass through damaged endothelial junctions into the brain itself. This allows more immune cells to leak into the brain, with T cells and macrophages being the most significant, causing escalating damage. This is an early process in the disease pathology of MS.

4. *Plaque formation* in the brain and spinal cord is an aspect of MS that progresses over time and disrupts the workings of the brain and its communication with the body, leading to progressive neurologic deficits.

5. According to a surge of new research,[3] the entire process of MS may be initially activated and then maintained by reactive oxygen species and oxidative stress leading to *apoptosis of cells*, including oligodendrocytes. Apoptotic material then overwhelms the brain's phagocytic ability (the ability of the cells to remove damaged cells or pathogens), causing local accumulation of damage to cells including damage to the venules, leading to leaky BBB. So oxidative damage, or *oxidative stress*, becomes one of the mechanisms of cellular damage and potentially the activating event, leading us to question the cause of the oxidative stress.

Lupus

Lupus is a complicated disease in which the immune system attacks, damages, and destroys the body's connective tissues and parts of its own DNA. It can affect many organ systems but especially affects the kidneys, joints, vasculature, and brain (neuropsychiatric disorders). It occurs mainly in women of childbearing age and is more prevalent in women of both African and Asian descent. But the presentation is so variant, and symptoms often so atypical, even for lupus, that many people go undiagnosed for years or decades, if they ever get the correct diagnosis at all.

While the pathological process of lupus is very complicated, it can be broken down into four major categories of pathology.

1. There are abnormalities in the activity of three main cells: B cell lymphocytes, T cell lymphocytes, and monocytes. One of the major self-perpetuating pathways that maintains the lupus disease process is a co-overstimulation between B cells and T cells in which B cell Ag presentation to the T cell HLA site causes excessive and uncontrolled T-helper cell activation which in turn activates B cells to overproduce, creating more self antibodies and immune complexes.

2. It is an inflammatory disease with excessive and imbalanced cytokine release. One such cytokine, interferon type 1 from dendritic

cells, stimulates the release of NETs (neutrophil extracellular traps), a dense spiderlike web that instigates further tissue damage and co-stimulates further immune complex formation.

3. It is a clearance disease in which there is an increase in cell death (apoptosis) and a decrease in the ability to clear the dead cells from the system. This is in large part due to abnormalities in phagocytic cells, especially dendritic cells and macrophages. Dendritic cells also release interferon type 1, which is highly inflammatory and activates more NET formation and therefore immune complex formation.

4. It is a type III hypersensitivity response, which means that B cells bind to a protein to form immune complexes that are deposited in the tissues, creating damage, especially significant in the kidneys, vasculature, joints, and connective tissue.

Current Known Causes and Treatments

Despite growing scientific knowledge about the pathological mechanisms of MS and lupus, the primary cause, or causes, that instigate and maintain the disease are still elusive. There are only three widely accepted contributing factors that are well-established for MS: vitamin D deficiency, smoking, and past infection with Epstein-Barr virus (EBV). Lupus can be drug-induced (usually resolves after the offending medication is stopped) and neonatal (usually transmitted from a mother who is in a lupus flare while pregnant or within six months of becoming pregnant). Other than these instances, both MS and lupus are said to be caused by unknown environmental factors in a genetically susceptible individual. The causes of MS and lupus—just what the "unknown environmental factors" are—are poorly understood.

Current medical treatments for both MS and lupus work by blocking some specific disease process, offering only improvements in symptoms without offering any modification of disease progression[4] and while carrying the risk of severe side effects. The problem with this approach is that MS and lupus are very complex diseases with many pathological mechanisms and cells involved. According to Dr. Rhonda Voskuhl, director of UCLA's MS program, the danger of targeting one molecule or one process of MS is that, due to the complexity of MS pathology, if you block one step in the disease process, others kick in and the disease just marches on.[5] This is the case with lupus as well.

While the factors that lead to the body's lack of tolerance to self are poorly understood, research over the last decade has shed new light on autoimmune diseases. This chapter is an extensive review of what research reveals about the activating factors of MS and lupus as well as real-world treatments that can improve response to therapy and quality of life. Low dose naltrexone (LDN) is highlighted as an important and inexpensive therapy that has profound effects on every step of disease instigation as well as the pathological processes that maintain it.

Genetics and Epigenetics

Genetics does not equal destiny. Genetic inheritance increases your risk of developing an autoimmune disease by about 20%–30%. A large part of the risk of autoimmune disease is due not to genetics, but to epigenetics. Epigenetics is the way your genetics are changed during your lifetime. There are many things that cause epigenetic changes leading to disease.

It is evident from research that autoimmune diseases are caused by an interplay between environmental influences leading to epigenetic changes that both instigate the disease process and determine responsiveness to therapy.[6] For many, epigenetics is hard to grasp, but it is the key to MS, lupus, and most autoimmune diseases and therefore must be understood before we can move forward. Research over the last several decades has firmly established that our genetics are modified and changed during our lifetimes. Every exposure to the environment—food, sleep, chemicals, hormones, stress, and even emotions—causes modifications to our cells and our genes.

In the case of MS, most of these genetic modifications are to the major histocompatibility complex (MHC) complex on T cells.[7] T cells are an important cell type of our immune systems that identifies and mounts an attack against foreign invaders (pathogens), and calls other cells of the immune system to help. The MHC complex is similar to a drive-up window in which other cells can attach to a T cell and give it information about what needs to be attacked. This is where the immune system seems to go wrong in MS—the T cells are activated toward the oligodendrocytes, the cells that make the myelin sheath around nerves.

According to Dr. Bruce Richardson, a researcher at the University of Michigan, the initial cellular trigger that sparks the ultimate development of lupus is oxidative damage. This in turn leads to an epigenetic change that inhibits DNA methylation in the T cells. This change to the T cells causes the conversion of T-helper (CD4) cells "into autoreactive, cyto-toxic, proinflammatory cells that cause lupus-like autoimmunity in mice and humans."[8]

Given that epigenetic changes are at the heart of autoimmune diseases, and given that environmental factors are the cause of epigenetic changes, there is significant cause for hope. If we can isolate the environmental triggers for epigenetic change, we can make choices that alter our genetics and disease progression in a positive way.

Naltrexone has been shown to decrease DNA methylation and other epigenetic changes induced in autoimmune diseases.[9] This makes the treatment of autoimmune diseases with LDN very significant as a proven therapy that potentially reverses some of the epigenetic changes that occur in autoimmune diseases.

The Environmental Factors

New research in the last decade indicates that interactions between the microbiome, epigenetics, and environmental triggers activate many disease processes, autoimmune diseases included.[10] Researchers have indicated that as much as 90% of the development of cancer and other diseases, especially chronic diseases, is due to diet and environment.[11] These and other studies indicate that autoimmune diseases are multifactorial diseases in which cells of genetically susceptible individuals are epigenetically modified by a combination of factors including one of two basic categories of triggers:

1. Gastrointestinal changes due to:
    A. Microbiome (all the millions of bacteria that live in our gut)
    B. Gluten and other food sensitivities
    C. Other dietary choices
2. Environmental factors including:
    A. Pathogens (viruses, bacteria, and other infectious agents)
    B. Nutritional deficiencies
    C. Chemical and environmental toxicity
    D. Endocrine (hormone) imbalance
    E. Sleep disturbance or deprivation
    F. Stress

THE GASTROINTESTINAL SYSTEM, OR GUT

It is easy to overlook the gastrointestinal system when talking or thinking about autoimmune diseases and, indeed, the gut has long been ignored in the research into the causes and treatment of MS and other autoimmune diseases. Some basic information on the gut puts us in the right frame of mind in relation to this misunderstood organ:

- 70%–80% of the immune system resides in the gut!
- The gut has more neurotransmitters than the brain, with some neurotransmitters being predominately located in the gut. For instance, 95% of serotonin, a common target of antidepressant therapy, is manufactured and utilized in the gut.
- The gut manufactures and uses more than twenty hormones that have both local and distant effects on organs such as the brain.[12] At least one bacterium in the human gut has even been discovered to produce androgens (male hormones).[13] All this makes the gut an important endocrine (hormonal) organ.
- Perhaps most obvious but also commonly overlooked, what we put in our mouths is of primary importance. All of the fuel and resources our bodies will ever get must be processed and absorbed through our guts. If we don't get the right building blocks, we can't build healthy cells. If we get toxins or poor nutritional content in our food, our hard cellular building gets torn down.

What, specifically, is happening in the gut of a person with an autoimmune disease? The microbiome refers to all the millions of bacteria that live in the gut. New research has implicated the gut microbiome as a causative factor in the development of MS. Dr. Sushrut Jangi, an instructor and researcher at Harvard Medical School, found an imbalance of the microbiome in MS patients such that an immune-enhancing bacteria is up to seven times more abundant in people with MS compared with controls, and immune-suppressing bacteria are three times less abundant.[14] A multi-center research study from Brigham and Women's Hospital[15] has shown similar results, with other bacterial imbalances that enhance and possibly instigate the autoimmune response. There is mounting research leading to the same conclusion: Changes in the gut microbiome are likely a significant trigger for development of MS.[16]

Furthermore, regional differences in diet, scientists have surmised, may lead to changes in the microbiome and explain the regional variation associated with MS risk. Researchers have also speculated that the difference in the microbiome between men and women is likely a major contributing factor to the significantly higher incidence of autoimmune diseases in women.[17]

Research published in 2014 makes the gut of primary importance in lupus and changes our basic understanding of this disease. It showed that epigenetic changes, *as influenced by the gut microbiome*, might be a significant trigger for the disease.[18] Before this time, the microbiome, and indeed the entire gut, had been largely disregarded in the pathogenesis of lupus. Now, however, based on this newer research, the gut and its microbiome are being investigated as major contributors to the development of lupus.

Making the gut–immune connection also explains some of the other triggers for autoimmune diseases in that the microbiome is influenced by diet, stress,[19] hormones,[20] environmental toxins,[21] exposure to pathogens, sleep, and medications, all of which are triggers for autoimmune diseases. The overlapping factors that both trigger autoimmune diseases and cause changes to the commensal bacteria in the gut make it a likely source of epigenetic changes leading to autoimmunity.

LDN has been shown in many studies to have positive benefits in immune diseases that center on the gastrointestinal system, such as Crohn's disease, ulcerative colitis, inflammatory bowel disease, and irritable bowel syndrome. These diseases and the improvement in the health of the gut and symptom improvement are covered elsewhere in this book. By decreasing the damaging inflammatory cytokines produced in the gut and altering the pathological cellular balance of autoimmune diseases, LDN supports the immune system to improve the balance of the microbiome.

GLUTEN

Gluten sensitivity is a common component of autoimmune diseases. Up to 80% of rheumatoid arthritis sufferers have gluten sensitivity and most autoimmune and in recent research many neurodegenerative conditions are being linked to gluten sensitivity. Professor Marios Hadjivassiliou, one of the most well-respected researchers in the area of gluten sensitivity and the brain at the Royal Hallamshire Hospital in Sheffield, England, reported in a 1996 article in *The Lancet*, "Our data suggest that gluten sensitivity is common in patients with neurological disease of unknown cause and may have etiological significance."[22] This statement is now being borne out in research with results indicating that the gut is potentially one of the most important triggers for the development of MS and other autoimmune diseases.

Research published in 2014[23] demonstrated that digesting gluten (found in grain) and casein (found in dairy) results in the release of peptides with opioid activity. These peptides cause changes to cystein methylation in the DNA, leading to epigenetic changes as well as having negative effects on glutathione and the overall oxidative burden in the brain. Gluten- and casein-containing diets lead to changes in the epithelial cells of both the gastrointestinal tract (leaky gut syndrome) and the brain (leaky BBB) via these opioid pathways.

In many people, gluten intake serves to initiate and potentiate the process of inflammation in autoimmune and neurologic disorders.[24] In fact, research in 2006 showed that gluten sensitivity can lead to lesions in the brain that could be confused with MS lesions on MRI scans.[25] And there are published case studies in which patients eliminated gluten and reversed the signs and symptoms of lupus entirely, prompting some doctors to call gluten sensitivity a masquerader of lupus.[26] Dr. David Perlmutter, an internationally recognized integrative neurologist, states in his book *Grain Brain* that he always checks patients for gluten sensitivity when they have been referred to him for MS and that he has found, "on many occasions," that patients' brain changes on MRI were in fact gluten sensitivity that created or mimic MS.[27] Dr. Perlmutter links the brain changes that are produced by gluten sensitivity to the development of a leaky BBB.

Dr. Alessio Fasano, a practicing gastroenterologist and researcher at Harvard Medical School, has shown that gluten intake leads to leaky gut syndrome in which normally excluded products, such as bacteria, yeast, pathogens, toxins, and partially digested foods, get absorbed through the damaged endothelial lining of the gut, activating the immune response to inflammation and autoreactivity.[28] He links these changes to a leaky BBB that develops when people with gluten sensitivity have gluten in their diets.

LDN has a positive benefit on the opioid pathways involved in the damage to the epithelial lining of both the gastrointestinal tract and the BBB. While removing gluten or dairy from the diet of the autoimmune patient can't be replaced by treatment with LDN, LDN is an important therapy that helps the gut to heal from these insults.

DIET

The standard diet of people who live in industrialized nations is loaded with sugar and refined carbohydrates, both of which raise blood sugar levels. When blood sugar is even mildly elevated it leads to glycation. The glycation process happens when sugar binds to proteins in the body. When this happens, it increases free radicals (oxidative stress) and inflammation. Glycated proteins, oxidative stress, and inflammation hyperactivate the immune system, causing changes in the microbiome leading to leaky gut syndrome. This in turn instigates a change in the BBB such that it becomes permeable, allowing immune cells access to the brain (where they should not be) as well as causing damage to the DNA. Once the T cells have entered the brain, they instigate the autoimmune attack against oligodendrocytes, the cells that make the myelin sheath surrounding the nerves.

Another dietary factor that has been shown to have a strong impact on MS development and disease progression is saturated fat. A thirty-four-year study followed MS patients who limited their saturated fat intake to below 20 g/day and those who did not. In the group that limited their saturated fat intake, there was a 5% mortality rate with average deterioration being reported as slight. Those who did not limit their saturated fat intake had serious disability and an 80% death rate over the period of the study.[29]

Research has shown that altering the gut bacteria with diet mitigated the symptoms of MS in mice[30] and many people have reported improvements in their MS symptoms with dietary changes. Dr. Terry Wahls is a physician with MS. She treated herself with a diet much like the paleo diet and has experienced significant remission of her symptoms. There has been a lot of controversy surrounding this doctor and her approach of treating MS patients with diet. However, it is prudent to explore any approach, especially one so simple and cost-effective, from which so many people have reported improvements in their symptoms and disease progression.

In some people, LDN changes the appetite, making it easier to stick with a diet that is low in carbs, sugar, and saturated fats. Research in mice and humans has shown that low doses of naltrexone have a positive benefit on dietary choices,[31] decreasing appetite and improving the ability to make healthier food choices.

PATHOGENS

There has been a long association between viruses, bacteria, yeast, and other pathogens and the development of autoimmune diseases. Studies have shown that when the body is fighting infection, cytokines that regulate sleep, as well as the HPA axis (discussed below), undergo changes[32] that may stimulate autoimmune diseases. One of the most important pathogenic causes of MS is an imbalance of the gut microbiome, as discussed above. But there are others.

Chronic Lyme disease is a pathogen that, like gluten sensitivity, has also been shown to have brain MRI results that resemble and are often mistaken for MS.[33] According to the National MS Society, Lyme disease can cause delayed neurologic symptoms and MRI findings that mimic MS, and can have a relapsing remitting or chronically progressive course once it develops. In a study published in 2000, researchers were able to show that 38.5% of people with MS had a positive serologic reaction to *Borrelia* (the pathologic organism in Lyme disease), which was twice the frequency of patients with other neurologic disorders.[34] This is especially significant because most people with chronic Lyme disease have false negative results on typical serologic testing.

Lyme disease is also another frontrunner to explain the regional difference in MS development in that "MS prevalence parallels the distribution of the Lyme disease pathogen *Borrelia* (*B.*) *burgdorferi*, and in America and Europe, the birth excesses of those individuals who later in life develop MS exactly mirror the seasonal distributions of *Borrelia* transmitting *Ixodes* ticks."[35] And while chronic Lyme disease has been downplayed in the Western medicine environment due to frequent false negatives with traditional testing, newer research has shown that chronic Lyme is in fact a real entity based on antibodies indicating long-term exposure to *Borrelia*.[36]

Epstein-Barr virus (EBV) is another pathogen that has long been linked to MS. People who have never had EBV (only about 5% of population) are at lower risk of developing MS. And if people contract EBV in adolescence or adulthood they are more likely to develop MS than if they contracted it in early childhood. However, the link between EBV and MS is unclear.

Several infectious agents have been so closely linked with lupus that it is not uncommon to see a paper begin with a statement that infections are known to trigger lupus expression and activity. Several potential pathological etiologies have been theorized to cause the activation of lupus in genetically susceptible individuals when exposed to multiple pathologic agents including viruses, bacteria, yeast and other fungi, parasites, and many infectious agents.[37] And it is viral proteins that inactivate the degradation of cellular DNA leading to immune complex formation.[38]

Research done at the Mayo Clinic in 2012 showed a link between chronic staph infections, even at very low levels, and the development of lupus.[39] Research has also shown that molecular mimicry to EBV can give rise to the disease process of lupus.[40] EBV titers have been shown to be up to forty times higher in people with lupus as compared to controls[41] and a reactivation of EBV with higher blood titers follows a lupus flare by about a week.[42] It can be theorized based on this and much more information defining the link between EBV and lupus that EBV also stimulates autoantibody production and abnormalities that contribute to the development, or progression, of lupus. Several other viruses have been implicated as triggers of lupus via mimicry, including cytolomegalovirus and parvovirus.[43] It seems clear from research that chronic infections contribute to the development of lupus.

LDN improves the immune system's response to infection. It has been shown in research to have a positive benefit in many types of infections, including HIV, herpes, hepatitis, and EBV. Patients with chronic infections of many types respond well to LDN with fewer, less frequent, and less severe infections, as well as improved response to therapy. LDN's positive benefits are likely due to its immunomodulatory effects on T cells, monocytes, and macrophages.

NUTRIENTS

There have been many studies regarding nutritional supplements that may help with MS, lupus, and other autoimmune diseases whether or not the patient is deficient in these nutrients (baseline blood levels are not even measured in most studies).

Nutrients and MS

Vitamin D deficiency is one of the three environmental factors known to increase the risk of developing MS. Patients who have vitamin D deficiency and already have MS are known to have a worse course for their disease and more relapses. Vitamin D deficiency is one of the leading theories for the geologic difference in MS risk, has been shown to decrease both the symptoms of MS and risk of developing MS in human and animal studies, and is known to have an immunomodulatory effect in MS.[44] In a study of patients who were in an active phase of MS, those given dosages ranging from 700 to 7,000 micrograms (mcg)/week had fewer enhancing lesions on MRI.[45] Vitamin D has been used at dosages as high as 40,000 IU daily for twenty-eight weeks followed by 10,000 IU daily for twelve weeks with a peak level of 413 nanomole (nmol)/liter (L) on blood work (100 nmol/L is usually considered the upper limit of acceptable) with no adverse outcomes and continued improvements in MS symptoms, fewer relapses, and improved T cell health.[46] Vitamin D has been shown to be a "biological inhibitor of inflammatory hyperactivity"[47] and vitamin D receptors have been found within the genome, implicating it as a factor in the epigenetic nature of autoimmune diseases.[48]

Vitamin D deficiency is also a potential explanation for the regional variation of MS. Humans convert vitamin D from sun exposure directly on our skin (when not wearing sunblock). People closer to the equator have lower rates of MS. They also have lower rates of vitamin D deficiency, which is rampant and more significant, as is MS, the further away from the equator you get. Vitamin D deficiency has been shown to increase the risk of developing autoimmune diseases through epigenetic dysregulation.[49] Vitamin D has also been shown in research to suppress the autoimmune reaction, to be especially beneficial in TH1-mediated autoimmune diseases (such as MS), and to actually prevent MS.[50]

Vitamin D is also implicated in the leaky BBB of MS. It is damage to the endothelial cells in the vasculature of the brain that leads to disruption of the tight junctions that maintain the BBB. Recent research showed that vitamin D deficiency led directly to more apoptosis of endothelial cells in vivo[51] (inside the human body) and treatment with vitamin D eliminated this effect.

Glutathione is the most important antioxidant in the CNS. Levels of glutathione are reduced in patients with MS and other autoimmune diseases, decreasing the brain's ability to deal with oxidative stress.[52] Alpha lipoic acid is a powerful antioxidant that easily crosses the BBB, increases levels of glutathione, and appears to have neuroprotective capabilities outstripping any medication currently available.[53] It has also has been shown to reduce the oxidative stress of MS. In mouse models it has been shown to decrease the ability of immune cells to cross the BBB into the brain, reduce the demyelination, and improve the health of neurons.[54]

In a five-week trial, glutathione increased by fivefold in patients given a combination of 6 mg sodium selenite, 2 g vitamin C, and 480 mg vitamin E a day. Antioxidant capability in MS patients is known to be lower than in people who do not have MS, contributing to or causing the increased oxidative damage that is a hallmark of the disease. Research has shown that taking antioxidants has a disease-modifying effect.[55]

Research has further elucidated that low-molecular-weight antioxidants may support cellular antioxidant defenses in various ways, including reducing oxidative stress, interfering with damaging epigenetic changes, reducing protein complexes, producing healthier enzyme activity, and producing metal chelation. Specifically, polyunsaturated fatty acids not only may exert immunosuppressive actions through their incorporation in immune cells but also may positively affect cell function within the CNS.[56]

High-dose biotin, another antioxidant, was shown to have a positive effect on symptoms, disease progression, and improvements in brain function over two years with onset of improvement of symptoms taking between two and eight months.[57] Dosages used in this study were 100–300 mg of biotin, levels that are unavailable over the counter, although they could be made at compounding pharmacies.

Melatonin has been found to have anti-inflammatory and immuno-modulating effects in the brain and have positive effects on many of the pathological processes in autoimmune diseases. It has also been shown to stabilize the endothelial cells of the vasculature, thereby improving the BBB distortions in MS.[58] Melatonin is worth a try to help improve sleep and may actually aid in the disease process itself. We know from research that it is safe to take dosages up to 20 mg nightly before bed.[59] I have my patients start at 1–3 mg before bed and increase until they sleep better, get to 20 mg, or must decrease due to nightmares or morning grogginess.

One research study to date has shown that administration of CoQ 10, a potent antioxidant, decreased disease progression and improved the pathologic mechanisms of MS in a mouse model.[60] I normally recommend ubiquinol (a better absorbed form of CoQ10), 200–400 mg daily.

Nutrients and Lupus

Vitamin D is also the most widely researched and understood nutrient associated with lupus. As much as 85% of people with lupus have vitamin D deficiency,[61] and research has shown that genes involved in autoimmune diseases and cancer are regulated by vitamin D.[62] Vitamin D levels have been shown to negatively correlate with disease markers and activity in lupus.[63] Vitamin D has been shown to mitigate autoimmune disorders by suppressing the autoimmune cellular activity and enhancing the TH1 immune pathway,[64] the imbalance of the TH1 and TH2 pathways being a significant part of the cellular pathology of lupus. Research has further shown that vitamin D promotes T cell regulation and inhibits effector T cells, which cause much of the cellular damage of lupus, and that this promotes tissue repair.[65] A study published in 2012 showed that lupus patients with low vitamin D levels (average 18 nanograms [ng]/deciliter [dL]) who were given high-dose vitamin D (100,000 IU weekly for four weeks followed by 100,000 IU monthly for six months) showed decreased T effector cell counts and autoantibodies and increased T regulatory cells. During the six-month follow-up of the patients in this study, no disease flares were noted.[66]

Although LDN has no direct effect on nutrient status, by contributing to repair of the gut lining, LDN likely improves nutrient absorption.

ENVIRONMENTAL TOXICITY

Dr. Sherry A. Rogers is a preeminent physician and researcher as well as a prolific writer of scientific papers and books. One of her specialties is environmental toxicity and detoxification. As she explains in her book *Detoxify or Die*,[67] and as the National Institutes of Health (NIH) has indicated based on environmental research over decades, we are bathed in toxins from the time we are in utero throughout all of our lives. In fact, research spearheaded by the Environmental Working Group in 2009 showed that ten randomly chosen newborn babies had, on average, 287 chemical toxins present in the umbilical cord on the day of birth.[68] Of those found, 180 cause cancer in humans or animals, 217 are toxic to the brain and nervous system, and 208 cause birth defects or abnormal development in animal tests.

According to the Chemical Industry Archives there are over eighty thousand chemicals in common use,[69] although the US Food and Drug

Administration (FDA) doesn't know what chemicals are currently in use nor what products they are present in, and most new chemicals (about 40–50 new chemicals every week) are not required to show any human safety information before they are approved. In fact, less than 5% of the chemicals that are currently abundant in our environment are tested for human safety. This is unforgivable given that exposure to chemicals has been implicated as the single instigating factor leading to autoimmune disease development.

According to the National Resources Defense Council (NRDC), clusters of autoimmune diseases have been reported all over the country. A disease cluster is defined as an unusually large number of people in a limited geographical area developing the same illness. The illness is usually caused by environmental toxins. In addition to the mounting scientific reports on these disease clusters, there are many more that are discovered but not reported or are reported to agencies that don't pursue investigation.[70] Scientists claim that this does not point to the particular toxins as being complicit in the cause of the disease since not all people who are exposed develop the disease in question. However, when we put the pieces of the scientific puzzle together, we see a very different story.

For example, in one literature report, Balluz and colleagues discovered higher-than-normal exposure levels to organophosphates and chlorinated pesticides in a community in Nogales, Arizona, where the prevalence of lupus in those residents is "two to seven times higher than the prevalence [of lupus] in the US population."[71] The normal prevalence of autoimmune diseases is about 5% of the population. If the prevalence of lupus in this community is two to seven times higher, that would make it between 10% and 35% prevalence. This exactly matches what genetics tells us—that about 20% to 30% of the population is susceptible to developing an autoimmune disease if exposed to the environmental toxins that can induce it.

MS has been associated with disease clusters in El Paso, Texas, that show elevated levels of lead, zinc, arsenic, cadmium, and suffer dioxide, and in Wellington, Ohio, that show evidence of chemical contaminants from a former foundry and an automotive parts manufacturer. Pesticides have specifically been shown to trigger MS in susceptible individuals in many studies.[72] Research and cluster studies have implicated many other xenobiotic organisms.[73]

Many other disease clusters involving autoimmune diseases have been reported.[74] The link between the development of immune system diseases (autoimmune diseases and cancer) and environmental exposure to toxins is so prevalent that the NRDC has called for better practices and a revision of the Toxic Substances Control Act. They also maintain a map of known disease clusters, although it is limited to those that have been officially investigated.[75]

There are many researchers who are exploring this aspect of disease induction and finding progressively more links indicating that environmental toxins are a potent instigator of disease. There is so much overwhelming proof of environmental toxins, and especially mercury, in the initiation or progression of lupus that even the NIH recognizes and reports this link between environmental toxins and lupus.[76]

Some of the known or theorized mechanisms by which environmental toxins trigger lupus or other autoimmune diseases are through mimicry,[77] endocrine disruption,[78] blocking the uptake of nutrients,[79] or activation or inactivation of epigenetic changes through oxidative damage.[80]

Environmental toxins have been shown to increase the production of autoreactive T cells and autoantibodies, stimulate the release of pro-inflammatory cytokines, and target end-organ damage.[81] Mercuric chloride (mercury) has been shown to cause immune complex glomerulonephritis in susceptible mice[82] and "mercury is also considered a potent immuno-stimulant and -suppressant, depending on exposure dose and individual susceptibility, producing a number of pathologic sequelae including lymph-oproliferation, hypergammaglobulinemia, and total systemic hyper- and hyporeactivities."[83] It is also known to be a potent toxin of the neurologic system causing brain symptoms such as fatigue, brain fog, memory issues, mood instability, increased risk of psychiatric diagnosis, and many more.

Mercury has been found to be able to bind glutathione,[84] the main antioxidant of the CNS, potentially reducing levels of glutathione available for use in the CNS. This would result in increased oxidative damage to the brain. In fact, lower glutathione levels have been documented in MS patients,[85] and this is an indication of oxidative stress. Oxidative stress has been implicated as a prominent triggering factor of both MS and lupus due to loss of antioxidant/oxidant balance.[86]

One of the ways in which environmental toxins have such a detrimental effect on some people even at relatively low exposures while having virtually no effect on other people with high exposure rates has to do with individual detoxification capacity. Most of the human body's ability to remove toxic substances is largely an aspect of the P450 enzymatic detoxification pathways through the liver, of which there are several hundred. These pathways contribute to disease in two ways: (1) there are dozens of known single nucleopeptide polymorphisms (SNPs), genetic variations that lead to a decreased detoxification capability of certain P450 pathways; and (2) the production of toxic intermediaries that overwhelm the ability of the body to clear the pathways.[87] SNPs are epigenetic changes that contribute to the development of autoimmune diseases.[88]

Several environmental toxins have been shown to inhibit P450 enzymes, including glyphosate, the active ingredient in Roundup and the world's most common herbicide. Research has shown that glyphosate's "interference with CYP enzymes acts synergistically with disruption of the biosynthesis of aromatic amino acids by gut bacteria, as well as impairment in serum sulfate transport" to cause insidious onset of inflammatory diseases throughout the body.[89] And this is only one of many chemicals we are all exposed to on a daily basis with known CYP 450 disruption.

People that have these SNPs can be referred to as "poor detoxifiers." They don't remove toxic substances from the system as well as the rest of the population. Researchers have estimated that up to 20% of the population may be poor detoxifiers.[90] When one is a poor detoxifier, environmental toxins can't be eliminated fast enough to match exposure rate and therefore toxins build up in the body, leading to disease onset through the mechanisms already mentioned above.

To understand this, one must understand the difference between acute and chronic toxicity. Acute toxicity is what can be tested through blood work. There is a false belief that toxins leave the system as soon as they are no longer at testable ranges in the blood. But as any specialist in chronic environmental toxicity will say, this is a misconception that gives both doctor and patient a false sense of security. A blood test is only indicative of recent exposure. Anything the body is exposed to today will be eliminated or stored within about two weeks' time. If it can't be eliminated, it must be stored in the tissues. Once it is stored in the tissues, it can remain there for a lifetime because the body is chronically re-exposed every minute of every day. Therefore, blood levels of toxins are only indicative of recent exposure and anything the body is releasing as cells die off or detoxify (from weight loss, rhabdomyolysis, nutritional and dietary factors, etc.). Chronic toxicity refers to toxins stored in the tissue and is therefore not testable through blood work.

LDN improves the body's ability to eliminate and manage toxic exposure in several ways. It improves glutathione levels, thereby aiding detoxification. It decreases oxidative damage caused by toxic exposure, making it easier for the body to clear the toxins. It decreases the autoreactive T cells and inflammatory cytokines that are a hallmark of environmental toxicity. It helps to repair the damage to the epithelial cells of the gut and BBB that is caused by toxins. And last, LDN helps to repair the toxin-induced DNA methylation that leads to epigenetic change.[91]

HORMONES AND THE ENDOCRINE SYSTEM

Elevations of estrogen and prolactin have been shown to increase the number of autoreactive B cells and to interfere with B cell tolerance.[92] Estrogen dominance (more estrogen than progesterone relative to one another in women and high estrogen levels in men, a term coined by Harvard physician John Lee) has been shown to activate inflammatory cytokines via the estrogen receptors on various immune cells associated with the development of autoimmune diseases.[93] Exogenous estrogens, nonhuman estrogen-like compounds found in industrial chemicals, pesticides, and surfactants, have also been shown to adversely affect the immune system and lead to development of autoimmune diseases through endocrine disruption.[94]

Hormones in MS

However, both estrogen and progesterone have been shown to be protective in MS. They have been found to dampen the brain's immune responses and regulate oligodendrocyte function.[95] Estradiol, the most active form of estrogen, has been shown to have an inhibiting effect on the overactive TH1 autoimmune pathway and to decrease inflammation in animal MS models via modulation of T cells.[96]

Part of the protective benefit of estrogen in women with MS may be due to a particular form of estrogen called estriol, sometimes referred to as the pregnancy hormone. It is well known that women usually have improvement in MS symptoms when they are pregnant. Research has shown that women treated with estriol had a decrease in enhancing lesions on brain MRI and decreased inflammatory cytokine production.[97] For estrogen levels in men with MS, though, there is a positive correlation between estrogen levels and brain damage.[98]

Regarding testosterone, both men and women with low testosterone levels have higher risk of developing MS and more progressive disease with more gadolinium enhancing lesions on MRI.[99] In a pilot study of ten men, researchers at UCLA showed that treatment with testosterone led to a disease-reducing shift of the immune cells, decreased inflammatory cytokine release, and increased release of growth factors that stimulate regeneration of the myelin sheath.[100] In 2011, Dr. Nancy Sicotte and colleagues at UCLA showed that giving men with MS testosterone had neuroprotective effects and was safe and well tolerated.[101]

The hypothalamus, pituitary, adrenal (HPA) axis has been shown to be impaired in people with MS.[102] Cortisol levels (a corticosteroid produced mainly in the adrenals) have been found to be lower than controls in MS brain lesions.[103] Levels of DHEA, a hormone secreted from the adrenal glands, are lower in people with MS.[104] DHEA deficiency has been shown to result in IL-2-deficient production from T cells (IL-2 has an immune-modulating effect) and replacing DHEA has been shown to improve IL-2 production.[105] Treatment with DHEA improves symptoms of fatigue. In seminal research at the Multiple Sclerosis Research Center at Vanderbilt University Medical Center, researchers showed that DHEA suppressed MS in an animal model.[106]

Dr. Voskuhl, at UCLA, stated in an interview that all the current disease-modifying therapies on the market today are designed to stop or slow down the immune attack but do nothing to halt disease progression.[107] On the other hand, she and her colleagues are working on hormonal neuroprotective therapies that would help to protect the brain from the autoimmune attack. She states that hormones have a neuroprotective benefit that could prove to have a marked decrease in permanent disability accumulation.

Hormones in Lupus

Research has shown that imbalanced hormones, especially estrogen dominance, DHEA deficiency, hypothyroid (even subclinical), and exogenous hormones (not coming from or relating to human hormones) all play a role in increasing the risk of developing or worsening the progression of lupus. But the body's natural hormones, when balanced, are protective. Patients who work to balance the endocrine system often experience improvements in the symptoms of lupus as well as slowing of the disease process.

One of the defects of lupus is that there is a decrease in the production of androgens (DHEA, testosterone), which has a mitigating effect on autoimmunity, and an increased production of estrogens, which enhances autoimmunity. There is also an increased conversion of androgens into estrogens in lupus patients and high levels of estrogens have been found in the joints of lupus patients.[108] Estrogen is known to be pro-inflammatory in nature whereas progesterone, androgens, and corticosteroids are anti-inflammatory.

Low levels of DHEA are found in most patients with lupus independent of corticosteroid therapy, and administration of DHEA has mitigated symptoms and decreased the need for corticosteroids.[109] Likewise, low testosterone levels are consistently found in women with lupus and administration of testosterone has resulted in clinical improvement of the disease. The same results were not found in men, but serum concentrations of estradiol and progesterone are not routinely measured in men, which may account for a lack of findings.[110]

Thyroid hormone is immune modulating in that people with lower thyroid production have higher rates of cancer, infectious diseases, and autoimmune diseases. Patients with lupus are more likely to have symptomatic thyroid problems and subclinical hypothyroid disease[111] and many of the symptoms of hypothyroidism overlap with lupus symptoms, namely fatigue, brain fog, memory, and sleep disorders. While there is no research evidence that hypothyroidism increases the risk of lupus, researchers have nonetheless called for frequent monitoring and early treatment of any thyroid derangements in patients with lupus.

Research has also elucidated part of the mystery of the gender difference in autoimmune diseases. A normally silent immune gene on the X chromosome is demethylated (this is an epigenetic change), making disease flares worse. Men must have a more robust trigger than women because they have only one X chromosome.[112]

LDN has a positive effect on the neurotransmitters in the brain. Research has shown LDN to be beneficial in depression, anxiety, and bipolar disorder. And it is known to help balance stress hormones.

LDN has a balancing effect on the HPA axis and all the body's hormones. This is the case because endorphins, the production of which are increased with LDN, have a controlling and directing effect on the immune and endocrine (hormonal) systems. Many patients have had resolution of their hormonal symptoms while taking LDN, and it is often prescribed just for this reason because it works so well.

SLEEP

Cytokines, hormones, and the HPA axis have all been shown to have an effect on sleep cycles.[113] Conversely, sleep has an effect on cytokines, the immune system, hormones, and the HPA axis. Sleep deprivation has been shown to be immunosuppressive,[114] potentially increasing the risk of infection and autoimmune activation. As well, the immune system is most active when we are in deep sleep, and poor sleep is the rule for most people who present with an autoimmune disease, making sleep an important factor in the development and maintenance of the autoimmune process. The body's detoxification processes and immune system are very active during sleep when your brain is resting. Since many people with an autoimmune disease may be poor detoxifiers or have genetic sensitivity to environmental toxins, deep restful sleep is very important for preventing disease flares as well as disease onset.

Sleep apnea is a special problem in which a person stops breathing due to obstruction from relaxation of the connective tissue in the throat (obstructive sleep apnea is most common) or from a lack of signaling from the brain (central sleep apnea). There is also a less severe but just as medically significant form called sleep hypopnea, in which the airway narrows without closing. Both sleep apnea and hypopnea can cause snoring, although the snoring may be so light that bed partners don't notice or don't complain. Both cause a block in the oxygen flow and therefore the oxygen levels in the blood drop, causing the sleeper to wake to a lighter level of sleep in order to open his or her airway and take a deep breath. This recurs from five to one hundred times an hour and keeps the person out of deep sleep.

Sleep apnea and hypopnea deprive the person of deep sleep needed for health maintenance and don't allow the immune system and brain the time they need for repair. Lack of deep sleep leads to dramatically increased risk of disease, and people with sleep apnea have many of the cytokine derangements that are present in lupus.[115]

Sleep apnea and hypopnea are poorly understood entities in our Western medicine society at this time. It is commonly believed that the only presentation of sleep apnea is in a grossly obese person who is snoring loudly enough to wake the whole house and is so tired that they fall asleep driving. And while this is common, I have diagnosed over one hundred patients who are at or close to their ideal weight with sleep apnea. Most of them were not loud snorers and didn't have the significant fatigue that would normally be expected from sleep apnea, otherwise they would likely have been correctly diagnosed before they came to me.

Research has shown that when an autoimmune attack is ongoing in the human body, cytokines that disrupt sleep are being produced.[116] LDN has a balancing effect on those cytokines that disrupt sleep. While the most common side effect of LDN is difficulty sleeping (about 20% of people who start directly on 4.5 mg experience this), most people sleep better and deeper and wake up feeling more refreshed with less daytime fatigue after tapering up to 4.5 mg, or whatever their stable dosage turns out to be.

STRESS

Acute stress is a powerful modulator of immune function.[117] In a 2011 *Neuroepidemiology* publication, Artemiadis and colleagues reviewed seventeen research studies that reported stress as a factor that potentially increases the risk of developing MS or of relapsing.[118] They found that fifteen of them showed a positive correlation. Research has further elucidated that while short-term stress may have some positive benefits, long-term stress causes an imbalance in hormones and neuromediators that results in down-regulation of protective immune system function and up-regulation of inflammatory pathways.[119] High stress for long periods of time increases abnormal cytokine production that mimics that seen in lupus patients in many ways,[120] leads to depletion of DHEA levels, and creates imbalances in the gut microbiome accompanied by damage to the lining of the intestines.[121] These abnormalities upset the balance of the immune system, creating a decreased ability to fight off disease.

LDN has been shown to reverse the cellular imbalances induced by chronic stress that contribute to disease. Multiple studies in rats have shown that pretreatment with naltrexone reduces the harmful cellular, immune, endocrine, and neurologic responses to stress.[122] Even neonates have been shown to benefit from treating pregnant rats with naltrexone in that it decreases the fetal response to stress.[123]

Treatment

There is never one thing that causes an autoimmune disease but rather a combination of triggering factors. In my practice, I have never seen an auto-immune patient who didn't have many of the triggering factors mentioned above. Additionally, many people have other triggers that aren't discussed in this chapter because although much circumstantial evidence exists, there isn't enough research to support scientific claims. On my first visit with autoimmune patients, I usually recommend extensive testing, appropriate to each person and tailored to their presentation. There are so many known risk factors that all of them should be ruled out. People seeking treatment will need to work with an integrative physician to accomplish this task.

Remember, there is no magic bullet. There is no one thing that works for every person with an autoimmune disease. This is where lay people and doctors alike get confused. But, for example, because dietary changes alone work for one person and not another doesn't make diet insignificant. It simply means that diet, the gut microbiome, leaky gut, and the concomitant changes, was the most significant activating factor in the person who responded to dietary changes and was not so in the person who didn't respond. Failing to see this is akin to the proverbial "throwing the baby out with the bath water."

If autoimmune diseases are due to epigenetic changes triggered by multiple environmental triggers, exploring all of these triggers is the key to a better life, slower disease progression, and, potentially, prevention in susceptible individuals.

The key to success with any treatment plan that requires patient participation is the patient's desire to do it. Desire is completely different from knowing one needs to do it, being required to do it, or feeling one should do it. None of those intentions will lead to success because the patient won't be able to maintain the required changes. He or she must truly want to do a thing in order to accomplish it. Desire, or drive, has long been known by successful people to be the key to success. The other required ingredient in a successful venture is persistent commitment to a goal. As the saying goes, "when the going gets tough, the tough get going." Patients have to develop their toughness to do combat with autoimmune diseases. So here's the plan of attack:

LDN

LDN has a worldwide following of patients who have experienced bene-fits in MS and lupus in that it both decreases relapses and prevents the progression of disease. LDN has been found to be so useful in so many people with MS that I would have to have an extremely good reason *not* to start it right away. Since LDN is now known to be safe in pregnant and lactating women[124] and to be of benefit for people who are on opioid pain medications,[125] even these need not be deterrents to therapy.

An Italian study of LDN that included 40 patients with primary progressive MS (PPMS) over six months showed that all but one had improvements in MS symptoms in this short time period.[126] LDN has likewise been shown to improve mental health and quality of life in MS patients.[127] Most studies have found LDN to be well tolerated with few dropouts and few adverse outcomes. I believe it is the ability of LDN to address many of the pathological biochemical processes that makes it so effective at improving symptoms and positively modifying the progression of autoimmune diseases.

Most MS patients can be started on LDN on their first visit. No labs need to be ordered. Some people even feel they are already noticing improvements within the first month of starting it. However, what people usually experience is a very slow improvement over months or even a period of a year or more. It can take as long as eighteen months to respond to LDN, according to some research and physician reports, so patience is the key to success with this treatment.

Specifically for lupus, LDN has been shown to enhance the deficient TH1 cell response[128] and balance the TH1/TH2 abnormality of lupus. It has a modulating effect on dendritic cells and a balancing effect on cytokine release,[129] decreasing inflammatory cytokine production. It helps to direct the immune system away from damaging, self-perpetuating pathways and back to healthier pathways of healing and repair. It helps to balance hormones, which is a very big factor in lupus. It helps people to sleep better as well, which is likely due to the balancing effect it has on the cytokines involved in sleep.

SMOKING

If an MS patient smokes, he or she must stop! People who smoke are more susceptible to MS and generally have more brain lesions and more brain shrinkage. Despite the health benefits to quitting smoking, nobody ever quits smoking, or anything else, until they are ready, no matter how dire their circumstances. There are some things that can help if a patient is committed to quitting smoking: acupuncture,[130] neurofeedback,[131] hypnosis (varying reports but works for some), counseling, or talking to a physician about medications.

DIET

"Let food be your medicine and medicine be your food." Or, as I like to tell my patients: Eat food that's just food. Our human bodies are built to digest food: plants, herbs, animals, fish, minerals. Just like we don't have the ability to digest rocks, bamboo, pine needles, and many other things, humans quite simply don't have the ability to digest exogenous hormones, chemicals, additives, preservatives, genetically modified organisms, or other nonfood entities without consequences to our health. We can put them in our mouths, true. But what happens after that can range from mildly irritating to progressively worsening or even to disastrous outcomes. It would be a mistake to disregard the importance of diet in overall health and especially in autoimmune diseases.

Regarding diet, start with what we know. Dramatically reduce or eliminate gluten, sugar, saturated fats, and all nonfoods. There is so much information about the benefits to the immune system with simple dietary changes that it would be foolish to overlook them.

- If patients are unconvinced about going GMO-free, have them watch the movie *Genetic Roulette*. That will change their mind.

- If patients are resistant to a gluten-free diet, test them for gluten sensitivity.

- If they have intense cravings for sugar that thwart their attempts to change their diet, they may have yeast overgrowth in their guts. Research has indicated that this change to the gut microbiota creates intense sugar cravings. *The Yeast Connection*, by Dr. William G. Crook, is a good book to read to help balance gut microbiota.

- Eliminating nonfoods, like most dietary changes, is easier said than done. As my grandmother used to say, "If you can't read it, don't eat it." Her sage advice proves much truer than I realized at the time. If there is an ingredient listed that isn't recognizable as an ingredient one would take off the shelf and add to food, put it back and look for something else. "Soy protein isolates" and other benign-sounding ingredients are code words for toxic substances that increase cravings for these foods. Food cravings are intense when these chemicals are first eliminated but die down over a two- to six-week period.

DETOXIFY

For the thousands of toxins that are not heavy metals and are known or suspected to contribute to the development of MS, treatment with far infrared sauna (FIR) therapy may be beneficial. There is currently an ongoing trial to evaluate this treatment modality that many people with immune system problems have found helpful. There are many books on detoxifying diets, supplements, foods, and lifestyle changes that will help accomplish the task of eliminating toxins from the body. Two of my favorites are *Detoxify or Die*, by Dr. Sherry A. Rogers (dramatic title, I know, but a very well-referenced scientific book), and *The Detox Diet for Dummies*, by Dr. Gerald Don Wootan. For removal of heavy metals, an integrative physician should appropriately test and treat patients.

HORMONES

Most female MS patients benefit from estriol with positive changes on MRI as well as symptom relief. Women should also be monitored for their balance of estrogen to progesterone on the twenty-first day of their cycle. During that time of the cycle, the estrogen/progesterone balance should be roughly 10/1. For example, if estrogen is 80, progesterone should be about 8 for the best balance. Progesterone is both anti-inflammatory and anti-proliferative and has been shown to have a positive impact on the progression of autoimmune diseases. Men should be checked for their estradiol, progesterone, testosterone, and dihydrotestosterone levels and balance them accordingly. Both men and women should have their thyroid and DHEA levels idealized. Working with a doctor who treats with bioidentical hormones is absolutely necessary.

SLEEP

I have never seen an autoimmune patient who was sleeping well on their first visit with me. I define good sleep as falling asleep within thirty minutes of going to bed, staying asleep throughout the night without waking (once is acceptable but not preferable), and waking up feeling rested. Someone who is waking more than once a night or sleeping less than seven uninterrupted hours a night is not getting enough sleep to support his or her immune system. Sleep deprivation is one of the factors that can trigger an autoimmune relapse and instigate the disease process if present in the context of other instigating factors. Don't just assume nothing can be done to improve sleep, especially if the only methods explored have been medications.

Neurofeedback is a neurophysiological treatment that has been researched and used in the medical community since the 1960s and is still utilized by NASA. It has proven benefit, researched over decades, in the treatment of insomnia and sleep disorders. There is more information and a list of local practitioners at this website: http://www.isnr.org (at the bottom, under "Resources," click on "Find an ISNR Member").

Melatonin has an immunomodulatory effect and decreases inflammation.[132] Other research has shown that melatonin has a balancing effect on the TH1/TH2 pathway,[133] so it's worth a try to help improve sleep and may actually help in the disease process itself.

Last and perhaps most important is treatment of sleep apnea or sleep hypopnea. I test all my patients who have more than one of the following symptoms: waking more than once a night (even to urinate), daytime fatigue, snoring (even lightly), startling or gasping awake, not being able to go back to sleep once they wake, blood pressure that requires more than two medications to manage or is still poorly controlled on medications, heart attack or stroke before the age of sixty or in a healthy person over the age of sixty, poor memory or brain fog, or persistent sleep problems despite their best efforts. I also test most patients in whom our attempts to treat sleep are unsuccessful, regardless of symptoms.

I use an unattended, or home, sleep study whenever possible. I believe I get more reliable results because people are in their own homes. The test is often covered by insurance and is so reliable that insurance companies will usually pay for treatment based on the results even if they don't pay for the test itself. Treatment for sleep apnea is not always a CPAP machine. In my practice, I rarely use CPAP, since at least 50% of my patients can't tolerate it. We usually go straight to APAP therapy. And patients with mild to moderate sleep apnea or with sleep hypopnea can be treated with an oral dental appliance or with EPAP therapy. Nearly all of my patients who have come in believing they couldn't tolerate treatment for sleep apnea are currently comfortable and happy on effective therapy. Patients should talk to a knowledgeable doctor about testing and, if appropriate, treatment options.

NUTRIENTS

The need for nutritional supplements should be tested as appropriate and nutrients should be supplemented in all people with an autoimmune disease, as indicated above in the nutrient-depletion section. There is very little risk of harm and big potential for improvement. Treatment must be consistent though, and the supplements used must be high quality.

STRESS

Although addressing stress can be the most difficult part of treatment for many reasons, not the least of which is the tendency to undervalue stress as an inducer of disease, research has so much to tell us about stress and disease induction or worsening that it is imperative to look at this aspect of treatment. I tell all my patients to do something every day to reduce stress: meditate, walk with a mantra (a short, positive sentence you repeat to yourself over and over—in my practice patients use, "Every day in every way I'm getting better and better"), read a book that helps them understand themselves or their world (a spiritual or self-help book), or read *Stop Worrying and Start Living*, by Dale Carnegie, which has techniques patients can use to get their stress under control.

There is an inexpensive way to learn to meditate. Brainwave research has brought us some interesting and powerful technologies that easily help to change the brain's unhealthy patterns. Listening to a CD or MP3 with binaural beats or hemispheric synchronization can decrease overactivity in the brain (findings on an EEG indicative of stress, worry, anxiety and inability to "turn off the brain") and help patients sleep better and reduce stress. Many of my patients have had success with this approach. There is even an inexpensive iPhone app called "Brainwave."

Summary

Low dose naltrexone has many positive benefits, both for modifying the disease processes of MS and lupus at the cellular level as well as for decreasing their symptoms. LDN can be used to improve sleep, balance hormones, improve the ability of the body to detoxify, help to stabilize epigenetic changes, improve the health of the gut, and modulate the immune response, changing immune pathways to healthier ones.

Talk to your doctor about LDN if you have an autoimmune disease or any disease associated with immune system pathology. You have nothing to lose and much to gain. Show your doctor this book—a conscientious physician wants to learn more to help their patients and will be glad for the scientific knowledge that will allow them to help you and many others. If your doctor is resistant to learning, resentful that you know something they don't, or tries to hamper your attempts to be healthy, please find another doctor. There are many compassionate physicians out there who are inquisitive, intelligent, and open-minded. There are many doctors who know that learning only begins with medical school, it doesn't end there.

But don't stop there. Explore all the known triggers of autoimmune diseases. Work with an integrative physician if you feel you're not making progress. Recognize what research is telling us: Our human bodies are complete systems that work together in harmony or disharmony. You must find all your contributing factors in order to optimize your health. Such are the requirements for a human body. I hope you find the journey toward health and recovery to be a rewarding one and that your life will be as healthy as possible.

THREE

Inflammatory Bowel Disease

Jill P. Smith, MD, FACP and
Leonard B. Weinstock, MD, FACG

Crohn's disease (CD) and ulcerative colitis (UC) share similar pathophysiology and approaches to medical therapy.[1] It is important to exclude other gastrointestinal disorders (such as irritable bowel syndrome, obstruction, celiac disease, and small intestinal bacterial overgrowth) prior to initiation of therapy for inflammatory bowel disease (IBD). Traditionally, treatment of Crohn's disease includes a variety of compounds designed to reduce the inflammatory response. Although 5-ASA compounds are very safe and remain the mainstay of therapy in UC, these agents used as monotherapy often do not maintain remission in ileal Crohn's disease. During acute attacks or flare-ups, corticosteroids augment conventional therapy, but these agents cannot be used for long-term maintenance due to systemic toxicity. For decades, thiopurines (azathioprine and 6-mercaptopurine) have been used to maintain remission in both CD and UC, and the availability of drug blood levels facilitates the management and decreases toxicity associated with these agents. Major advances in the understanding of the pathogenesis of IBD have led to the development of novel therapies called biologics. Such treatments include the administration of monoclonal antibodies specific for molecules expressed by the T cell population[2] or antibodies specific for cytokines known to be central to the pathogenesis of mucosal inflammation (i.e., anti-tumor necrosis factor, anti-TNF).[3] Unfortunately, treatment with many of these agents often leads to serious side effects.[4] Among the serious adverse events are the development of serious opportunistic infections and neoplasms,[5] and in children or young adults a fatal condition called hepatosplenic lymphoma has been reported.[6] Many patients with IBD have partial response or difficulty maintaining remission to medical therapy with single agents, and additional treatments are often required.[7] Unfortunately, still about half the patients do not achieve remission with the biologics and many develop resistance over time as the result of development of antibodies to the biologic protein. When immunosuppressive medications like thiopurines are combined with biological therapy ("combination therapy") there is a reduction in IBD flare-ups, a decrease in corticosteroid dependence, and a greater incidence of remission.[8] When combination therapy is not satisfactory, there are several concerns and options. To determine if medications are failing, it is wise to check therapeutic levels and antibody levels to assist in adjusting doses, changing to a different immunomodulator, manipulating thiopurine levels with allopurinol, switching to a different biologic agent, or adding adjunctive therapy.

Commonly used adjunctive therapies include antibiotics, probiotics, restricted diets (elemental liquids, gluten-free, FODMAP-free, and, rarely, total parenteral nutrition). Because of the toxicity and inadequate efficacy of the immunosuppressive and biologic medications used for IBD, novel strategies that are safer are desirable.

The standard approach to IBD is to alter inflammatory pathways in the intestinal lining, suppress the immune system, and administer antibodies against pathogenic antigens. These approaches all have risks to the patient. Treatment with prednisone or narcotic analgesics and an increased age are associated with increased mortality.[9] Factors independently associated with serious infections included moderate-to-severe disease activity, narcotic use, prednisone, and anti-TNF-α treatment. Suppression of leukocyte activity by steroids or bone marrow suppression as a complication of immunosuppressants places a patient at risk for bacterial infections.

Opioid Receptors and Pathophysiology of IBD

Both diseases start as mucosal diseases, although CD can involve the entire gastrointestinal tract while UC involves only the colon. Crohn's disease can start with shallow ulcers or erosions and later advance to deep ulcers that create fibrous tissue and strictures of the intestine. Penetration of the intestine by deep ulcers leads to abscess formation or fistulas. The pathways of inflammation for CD and UC have various similarities.

The mu-opioid receptor has been evaluated in the small bowel and colon, isolated peripheral blood mononuclear cells and purified monocytes, and

CD4[10] and CD8[10] T cells from healthy donors and IBD patients.[10] The effect of cytokines and nuclear factor kB (NF-kB) activation on the mu-opioid receptor expression in lymphocyte T and monocytic human cell lines was assessed. A synthetic mu-opioid-receptor agonist called DALDA (D-Arg[2], Lys[4], dermorphin-(1,4)-amide), which has been found to induce anti-inflammatory effects, was investigated in mucosal tissue samples from controls and IBD patients.

The mechanism by which opioid receptors influence inflammation is not clearly understood in IBD. Classical opioid receptors are categorized into three major types, mu, delta, and kappa, with delta receptors again divided into delta-1 and delta-2 subtypes. These receptors bind endogenous peptides, such as enkephalins and endorphins, as well as synthetic opiates such as morphine and its derivatives. Endogenous enkephalins bind to both the mu and delta receptors, although not to the kappa receptor, but they have higher affinity for the delta-receptor class. In addition, opioid receptors display a basal or constitutive activity even in the absence of ligand.[11] Opioid receptors are members of the rhodopsin-like family of G-protein-coupled receptors (GPCRs) and can form homo- or hetero-dimers as well as interact with other cell surface receptors, including chemokine receptors.[12] Likewise, cytokines and chemokines are small proteins that also interact with distinct GPCRs to act as integrators of inflammation.[13] Evidence is increasing that opioids regulate immune responses in part through their effects on cytokines and chemokines and their receptors.[14] While the immunomodulating activity of opioids is not fully understood, several recent papers have demonstrated that the heterodimerization between opioid receptors and chemokine receptors can both positively and negatively affect their activity. In fact, receptor heterodimers can have pharmacological properties distinct from either monomers or dimers of the parent receptors. Pello and colleagues have shown that interactions between the chemokine CXCR4 receptor and the delta-opioid receptor lead to the suppression of signaling of both receptors. However, Parenty and colleagues demonstrated that heterodimers of the delta-opioid receptor and CXCR2 chemokine receptor enhanced delta-opioid receptor function in the presence of the CXCR2 ligand.[15] Interestingly, although this report did show that ligands for CXCR2 modulated delta-opioid receptor function, they did not test the effect of delta-opioid receptor agonists or antagonists on chemokine-receptor function. The mechanism by which delta-opioid-/chemokine-receptor heterodimers exhibit their distinctive signaling properties is still under investigation. Others have shown that the mu-opioid receptors cross-talk with chemokine receptors by a mechanism termed heterologous desensitization.[16] It is thought that the desensitization occurs by phosphorylation and internalization of the opioid receptors.[17] Both opioids and opioid receptors are normally expressed throughout the gastrointestinal tract, and the expression of these receptors can increase during inflammation.[18]

Other signaling pathways downstream of G-protein activation may also be involved in cellular responses to opioid binding. Naltrexone, being a nonselective antagonist, interacts with all three receptor subtypes: mu-, delta-, and kappa-opioid receptors. Zagon and colleagues have proposed that naltrexone may act through a unique opioid receptor called the opioid growth factor receptor, or OGFr, that unlike the classic mu, kappa, and delta receptors is located not on the plasma membrane but on the nucleus of the cell.[19] The major ligand for this receptor is [Met]^5-enkephalin, and when it interacts with this receptor, cellular growth is inhibited. Zagon and colleagues showed that low dose naltrexone (LDN) could heal ulcers of the cornea by interacting with the OGFr and stimulating corneal growth and tissue repair.[20] Because of its role on the OGFr, Smith and Zagon postulated that LDN could have a similar effect on healing ulcers in the colon associated with ulcerative colitis and Crohn's disease. One mechanism by which [Met^5]-enkephalin is proposed to act is by stimulation of T cell proliferation through crosstalk and activation of the MAP kinase pathway.[21] Recent work on the role of [Met^5]-enkephalin and immune cells showed that this peptide modulates various lymphocyte populations to regulate immune responses.[22]

Role of Endorphins in IBD

Neuropeptides may play a role in IBD, and these molecules, which include enkephalins and endorphins, are present in the gastrointestinal tract and help modulate immune responses.[23] Up-regulation of [Met5]-enkephalin (also called "opioid growth factor" or "OGF") and opioid receptors and increased levels of endorphins can be induced by a rebound effect from administration of the short-acting LDN.[24] LDN will temporarily displace endogenous endorphins bound to the opioid growth and endorphin receptor. The up-regulation phenomenon is marked by these cells becoming temporarily deficient in OGF, which results in a rebound in receptor production. Receptor sensitivity is increased to capture more OGF and production of OGF is also increased to compensate for the perceived shortage of this molecule.[25] These levels of endogenous opioids inhibit cell proliferation, which then suppresses B and T lymphocyte responses.[26]

In an animal model of colitis, naltrexone reduces the inflammation by decreasing tissue pro-inflammatory interleukins 6 and 12.[27] There are opioid receptors on all inflammatory cells[28] and endorphin modulation via the mu-opioid receptor may have direct consequences in reducing inflammation.[29] In another animal model, prolonged activation of the toll-like receptor allows for increase in bacterial translocation and the negative effects may be expected from enhanced long-term administration of exogenous opioids (which suppress the endogenous opioid system).[30] Too much activation of the mucosal toll-like receptors may play a role in IBD.[31] Naltrexone can bind directly to toll-like receptors on macrophages in the central nervous system[32] thus decreasing inflammation. If naltrexone binds briefly to mucosal toll-like receptors this may improve host protection against microbial organisms on the intestine.[33] An up-regulated endogenous opioid system with OGF might have positive effects on the toll-like receptors.

LDN in Crohn's Disease

Starting in 2007, research has been published showing that LDN is beneficial in adults with CD.[34] This important pilot study, by Dr. Jill Smith and colleagues, demonstrated clinical response and even closure of fistulas in several patients. Subsequently, a randomized, placebo-controlled, double-blinded study demonstrated efficacy with naltrexone showing evidence for symptomatic, endoscopic, and histologic improvement compared to controls.[35] Preliminary studies in children with CD also suggest that there is safety and efficacy of LDN in this population.[36]

In Smith and colleagues' adult Crohn's disease randomized, placebo-controlled study, naltrexone was also used as adjunctive therapy (although biologic therapy was an exclusion for enrollment).[37] The results of this study showed that 88% of the naltrexone group (N=18) had at least a 70-point decrease in CD activity index scores compared to 40% of the placebo group (N=16). After twelve weeks, 78% of the naltrexone group had a significant response in the Crohn's disease endoscopy index severity score (CDEIS) compared to a 28% response in the placebo controls; 40% of the naltrexone group had endoscopic remission with CDEIS scores less than 6, compared to 0% of the placebo group. Biopsies were obtained from patients undergoing colonoscopies and scored for inflammation by a pathologist who was unaware of the treatment. There was no change in the inflammation scores over baseline scores in those subjects on the placebo; however, significant improvement with less microscopic inflammatory cells in the biopsies was observed in the naltrexone-treated patients compared both to their baseline scores (p<0.05) and to placebo-treated patients (p<0.0001). This study was the first double-blinded randomized controlled study to show improvement with a treatment (naltrexone) using histologic biopsies.[38] Although this clinical trial was not compared head-to-head with a biologic agent, endoscopic remission rates and clinical benefit from naltrexone was very similar or better than that described using anti-TNF-α agents. Furthermore, more than half of the patients in Smith and colleagues' naltrexone trials had already failed or had adverse reactions to biologic agents and were deemed to represent a more severe population and drug-resistant group with CD.

At the 2015 American Gastroenterology Association meeting in Washington, DC, results from 56 subjects treated long term with LDN for CD were presented.[39] Two-thirds of the patients in this study experienced either complete or partial remission by the Harvey-Bradshaw index. These results are supportive of the potential use of LDN to treat subjects with active CD who are not responding or achieving remission with standard regimens.

LDN in Ulcerative Colitis

Since LDN has been shown to clinically improve Crohn's disease, there was reason to believe it would also be efficacious in ulcerative colitis, the other major inflammatory bowel disorder. Several anecdotal reports have been cited, but large placebo-controlled trials have not been done in UC. Typically in my clinical practice LDN has been offered to UC patients who were failing standard medical therapy that included biologics. With respect to comparison to prior research in IBD, anti-TNF agents were not allowed in Smith and colleagues' CD studies, since patients tend to have worsening of symptoms prior to infusions and it was determined to eliminate this potential variation that could interfere with determining response.

Cases of Ulcerative Colitis Where Naltrexone and Biologics Were Combined

A female patient with UC who was becoming progressively worse with frequent diarrhea, bleeding, and cramps was treated with LDN. She experienced an initial response to infliximab, but this therapy became less effective over time. With the addition of LDN to her infliximab therapy she had a marked clinical improvement, which corresponded to mucosal improvement that was substantiated by colonoscopy. This patient was subsequently changed to adalimumab and naltrexone was continued. For over six years she has remained in remission except for one occasion when she stopped LDN on her own. Reinstitution of the LDN led to remission. This patient represents an example of combination of naltrexone with biologics where naltrexone therapy was effective and led to remitting disease.

Case Review Series

In a review of patients who had been treated with LDN for UC, an open-label study with long-term follow-up suggestive of benefit in UC patients was published.[40] The findings of this study included twelve case studies.

Patient 1: A forty-five-year-old man with a twenty-five-year history of UC was in clinical and endoscopic remission for over six years on 5-aminosalicylate therapy until September 2011. At that time he was admitted to the hospital for bloody diarrhea. Colonoscopy showed severe colitis (figure 3.1a), biopsies showed active colitis, and fecal studies were negative for an infectious etiology. The patient responded well to addition of intravenous methylprednisolone and increasing the 5-aminosalicylate dose. Slight tapering of high-dose prednisone led to recurrent bleeding and joint pain. In the distant past, 6-mercaptopurine was terminated owing to elevated liver chemistries. Infliximab was started in October 2011 and 5-aminosalicylate was continued. The patient went into a clinical remission that lasted for nine months. In July 2012 he developed progressively worsening low-grade fevers, joint aches, and bloody diarrhea. In December 2012, naltrexone 4.5 mg/day was added to his regimen. The patient had a prompt response in all symptoms within a month. Colonoscopy was repeated in March 2013, and there was complete mucosal and histologic healing (figure 3.1b). As of his last clinical follow up in April 2015 he has had no symptoms consistent with active IBD and remains on 5 mg/kg infliximab every eight weeks, 5-aminosalicylate 2.4 gm/day, and naltrexone 4.5 mg/day.

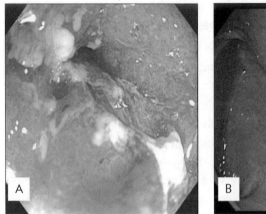
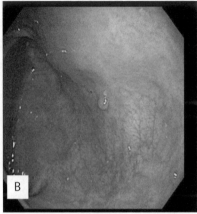

FIGURE 3.1. *A*, Severe ulcerative colitis with marked edema, erythema, and mucopurulent material on the surface. *B*, Remission in the ulcerative colitis after the addition of LDN—a small pseudopolyp is visualized along with atrophy and chronic vascular changes.

Patients 2–12: A summary of the clinical data for the 11 other patients treated with LDN is included in table 3.1. In total the 12 patients received naltrexone 4.5 mg/day as adjunctive therapy when biologic therapy (N=7), mercaptopurine (N=6), combined therapy (N=3), and prednisone (N=2) failed to control UC symptoms. One patient dropped out owing to insomnia as an adverse event after eight weeks and is counted as a treatment failure. Six of 12 patients reported moderate to marked improvement. Clinical responders continued naltrexone for 69 ±88 weeks.

The outcome of these UC colitis patients was similar to the same author's experience seen in his CD patients who failed conventional therapy.[41] At the time of this 2014 publication, a chart review was performed in 33 CD patients with moderate to severe disease who had been treated with naltrexone 4.5 mg/day as adjunctive therapy over a mean of forty weeks. With regard to side effects, 5 patients stopped therapy owing to adverse events—these were included in the treatment-failure group. Virtually all of these adverse events were insomnia and these mild to moderate adverse events rapidly improved with cessation of therapy. Preliminary evidence of efficacy determined by self-assessed questionnaires (as defined for the UC patients above) showed that 15 of the 33 (46%) had a positive clinical response and 18 of the 33 (54%) failed therapy. Of the 15 clinical responders,

11 had colonoscopy or ileoscopy before and after addition of naltrexone: 8 of the 11 had complete mucosal healing, 1 of the 11 had partial mucosal improvement, and 2 of the 11 were unchanged. These results suggest that naltrexone therapy is also efficacious in patients with UC.

Naltrexone: Drug Information and Side Effects

Naltrexone carries a warning from the FDA for hepatotoxicity at high doses. Two subjects in the CD placebo-controlled trial[42] developed a transient increase in liver enzymes while taking the low dose (4.5 mg) of naltrexone, but both resolved spontaneously without discontinuing the medication. Because of the risk for liver toxicity, it is recommended to not use this medication in those with known liver disease and to monitor liver transaminases periodically (every three to six months) while on LDN. According to the FDA, there have been no reported cases of withdrawal reactions when stopping naltrexone and none were reported in any of the clinical trials or case reports. It is not necessary to taper the medication when discontinuing the drug. Since naltrexone is an opioid-receptor antagonist (blocker) it will also interfere with narcotic analgesics, drugs such as codeine or morphine. Alternatively, these narcotic opiates may also interfere with the action of naltrexone; therefore these narcotic analgesics are not recommended while taking naltrexone. Since naltrexone is FDA-approved for alcohol withdrawal syndromes, naltrexone may interfere with the overall well-being or euphoria people experience from alcohol consumption.

Since naltrexone is water-soluble and crosses the blood brain barrier, it is thought to possibly interfere with endorphins and result in insomnia or induce vivid dreams. In the CD studies approximately 10% had insomnia. In the double-blind adult study however,[43] sleep disturbances were common in both naltrexone and placebo, suggesting that perhaps insomnia was a common condition in those with CD rather than due to the therapy. The only adverse event that showed statistically significant difference between the groups in the double-blind study was fatigue, which was more common in placebo-treated subjects.[44] In one review of a large group of patients, LDN-induced adverse events had rapid improvement with cessation of therapy and these events were mild to moderate in severity.[45] Changing the timing of LDN administration to the morning may reduce the incidence of insomnia. Gradually increasing the dose from 1.0 mg/day to 4.5 mg/day may also be helpful in those experiencing side effects, but may also slow the response and may not be necessary in most cases. In contrast to the standard therapies with immunomodulators, corticosteroids, and biologics used for IBD, naltrexone did not suppress the immune system or increase the risk for infections. Therefore, the safety profile for this compound is very good.

Dosing of Naltrexone

The dose of naltrexone used in the IBD subjects was 4.5 mg/day and this dose was selected based upon studies done on mice with chemically induced colitis that showed reversal of inflammation, reduction in tissue cytokines, and improved clinical activity only with a low dose and not a high dose of naltrexone.[46] One hypothesis regarding the mechanism of action of naltrexone at the low dose is related to its shorter interaction with the opioid receptors. If low dose (i.e., 4.5 mg or less per day) of naltrexone is given, the receptors are blocked for up to six hours (figure 3.2). During this time the body responds by releasing more endorphins and enkephalins, but these endogenous peptides cannot interact with the opioid receptors since naltrexone is occupying the

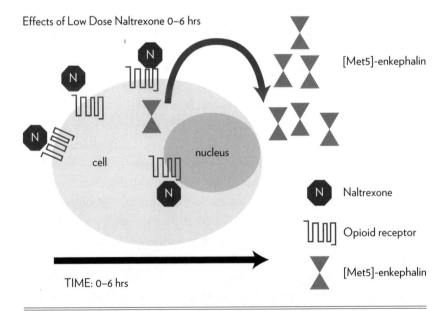

FIGURE 3.2. Proposed mechanism of a low dose of naltrexone. When a low dose of naltrexone is given, it is hypothesized to block the opioid receptors for only 0–6 hrs. During this time the cells respond by increasing endogenous blood [Met5]-enkephalin (OGF), but the receptor is blocked so the OGF has no effect.

Effects of Low Dose Naltrexone 6–24 hrs

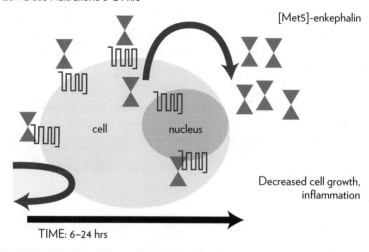

[Met5]-enkephalin

cell

nucleus

Decreased cell growth, inflammation

TIME: 6–24 hrs

FIGURE 3.3. Proposed mechanism of a low dose of naltrexone. After the low dose of naltrexone has been metabolized and excreted, it no longer blocks the opioid receptors and [Met5]-enkephalin (OGF) can now act on the receptors to down-regulate cell proliferation and inflammation. This hypothesis assumes that the naltrexone is no longer in the system and that the OGF levels are still elevated.

Risks If Naltrexone Dose Is Too High

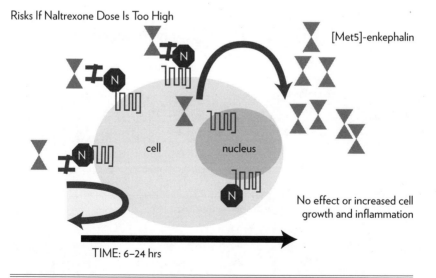

[Met5]-enkephalin

cell

nucleus

No effect or increased cell growth and inflammation

TIME: 6–24 hrs

FIGURE 3.4. Risks if naltrexone dose is too high. If the naltrexone dose is too high, then the opioid receptors will remain blocked for longer than 6 hours and up to 24 hours (at the 50 mg/day dose), and [Met5]-enkephalin is unable to interact with the receptor.

receptor site. After about six hours, the LDN is metabolized and no longer binds to the opioid receptors (figure 3.3). Now the elevated enkephalin or endorphins can interact with the opioid receptors to block cell proliferation or reverse inflammation. If however, naltrexone is administered at a higher

TABLE 3.1. Clinical Characteristics and Outcome of the Twelve Ulcerative Colitis Patients Treated with LDN as Adjunctive Therapy When Conventional Therapy Was Failing

Patient no. (Gender/Age)	Infliximab (IFX)	Mercaptopurine (6MP)	Prednisone (Pred)	5-aminosalycy-lates (5ASA)
1 (M/45)	1	Failed or had AE from mercaptopurine		1
2 (F/38)	1	1		1
3 (F/50)	1	Failed or had AE from mercaptopurine		
4 (M/25)	1	1		1
5 (M/60)	1			1
6 (M/53)	1			1
7 (F/21)	1	Failed or had AE from mercaptopurine		
8 (M/56)	1	1	1	1
9 (F/70)	Allergic reaction to infliximab	1		
10 (F/42)		Failed or had AE from mercaptopurine		1
11 (M/31)	1	Failed or had AE from mercaptopurine		1
12 (F/35)		Failed or had AE from mercaptopurine	1	1
Mean ± Standard error of the mean (SEM)				
43 ± 16 yrs	7	6	2	9
48 ± 76 wks	3	3	6	1

* Low dose naltrexone 4.5 mg daily

† LDN failure included those not helped, temporarily or slightly helped, or those who withdrew owing to an AE.

dose, such as the 50 mg/day dose used to treat alcohol withdrawal syndromes, then naltrexone occupies the opioid receptors for twenty-four hours (figure 3.4), and although enkephalin may be increased, this peptide cannot interact with the blocked receptor to exert an effect.

Low Dose Naltrexone (LDN) use (wks)*	Marked improvement	Moderate improvement	LDN failure†	Adverse event (AE)
32	1			
270	1			
6			1	
8			1	
8			1	1
8		1		
105	1			
24			1	
54		1		
28			1	
8			1	
6		1		

Based upon the hypothesis that LDN exerts its effect by transient opioid-receptor blockade and subsequent elevation in endogenous enkephalins and endorphins, using a cell-culture model system Donahue and colleagues showed that intermittent treatment with naltrexone, but not continuous therapy, resulted in the same effect as applying enkephalin to the cells.[47] In this cell-culture model that used cancer cells, the researchers also showed that continuous blockade of the opioid receptors by naltrexone (high dose) stimulated cancer growth. Because of the potential of stimulating cancer growth at high dose in someone with an existing malignancy, the high-dose therapy is not recommended and may have untoward effects.

Conclusions

This chapter summarizes the literature regarding the use of LDN in two inflammatory bowel disease states: Crohn's disease and ulcerative colitis. In both situations, LDN has promoted mucosal healing, decreased inflammatory activity, and improved quality of life. Furthermore, LDN has been administered in conjunction with immunomodulators and biologics where its concomitant use was clinically beneficial and without additional side effects for extended periods of time. The interaction of LDN with inflammatory cells and chemokine receptors may help explain its role in mediating response to inflammatory states. One possible mechanism of action for LDN includes the transient occupation of the opioid receptors, which up-regulates the endogenous enkephalin and endorphins that subsequently influence cell function and inflammation, has been proposed. Other mechanisms have also been examined, including the blockade of toll-like receptors on microglial cells to decrease neuroinflammation and pain. Others have shown that naltrexone has preferential binding to certain opioid receptors at the low dose (i.e., to the delta and OGF receptor rather than the mu receptor). Further studies are needed using LDN in IBD since all but two of these studies were double-blinded and the numbers of patients were relatively small. Double-blind studies are required to make any firm conclusions regarding likelihood of responding to therapy, since there is a high-placebo response seen in IBD.[48] The potential benefits of using a medication of low toxicity and good clinical efficacy is exciting.

FOUR

Chronic Fatigue Syndrome and Fibromyalgia

Kent Holtorf, MD

Chronic Fatigue Syndrome (CFS) and fibromyalgia (FM) are disabling conditions that are shown to be present in 0.5%–5% of the population and often coexist. Treating CFS and FM patients is often frustrating for physicians, as there is no clear etiology or treatment, and the use of standard recommended treatments that don't address the underlying pathophysiology, including nonsteroidal anti-inflammatory drugs (NSAIDs), antidepressants, and muscle relaxants, are largely ineffective and have significant side effects. Reliance on these medications results in a poor prognosis and is unsatisfying for both patients and physicians. It is unlikely that there is a single causative agent or process occurring in these conditions; therefore, a simple prescription is not likely to prove totally effective.

Many physicians and lay people consider CFS and FM to be "wastebasket" diagnoses, because the diagnoses have nothing to do with the underlying etiologies. Many dismiss these conditions as psychiatric in nature.[1] This does a disservice to the estimated 4%–7% of the population who suffer from these conditions. These disorders, which strike women four times as often as men,[2] are consistently associated with a unique set of physiological abnormalities, a hallmark of which is immune dysfunction.[3] Based on a comprehensive set of blood work alone, we can, without exception, differentiate those who suffer from CFS or FM from those who don't with about 70%–80% accuracy, without a history or physical (which are usually responsible for 80%–90% of the diagnoses). Furthermore, we can also consistently determine the likely severity of the condition as well as predict the underlying cause of the disorder by assessing the relative dysfunction of the ten to fifteen basic systems of the body.

Definition and Diagnosis of CFS and FM

A comprehensive review is beyond the scope of this chapter, but the most important underlying abnormality in these conditions is immune dysfunction. This immune dysfunction can be caused by a multitude of physiological insults, including infections, stress, toxins, and other causes of inflammation (figure 4.1). This then causes a vicious cycle of increased inflammation, which in turn causes further immune dysfunction. While standard medical practices focus on the infectious side of the vicious cycle, new research shows that better outcomes may be obtained with dramatically fewer side effects by focusing on the immune system. Additionally, many clinicians and experts in the treatment of CFS and FM are realizing that even if an underlying infectious cause is detected, unless the other half of the vicious cycle, the immune system, is addressed, long-term benefits are unlikely to be obtained.

The Centers for Disease Control and Prevention (CDC) definition of chronic fatigue syndrome (CFS) (recently renamed "systemic exertion

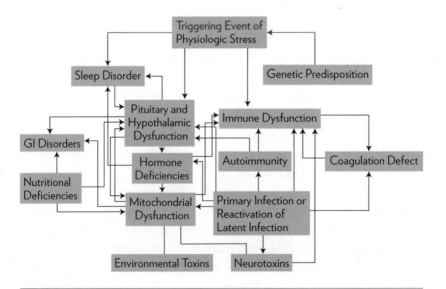

FIGURE 4.1. Causes of Immune Dysfunction

intolerance disease," or SEID), is the presentation of clinically evaluated, unexplained, persistent, or relapsing chronic fatigue that is of new or definite onset (has not been lifelong); is not the result of ongoing exertion; is not substantially alleviated by rest; and results in substantial reduction in previous levels of occupational, educational, social, or personal activities. Patients must have concurrent occurrence of four or more of the following symptoms, all of which must have persisted or recurred during six or more consecutive months of illness and must not have predated the fatigue:

- Self-reported impairment in short-term memory or concentration severe enough to cause substantial reduction in previous levels of occupational, educational, social, or personal activities
- Sore throat
- Tender cervical or axillary lymph nodes
- Muscle pain
- Multijoint pain without joint swelling or redness
- Headaches of a new type, pattern, or severity
- Unrefreshing sleep
- Postexertional malaise lasting more than twenty-four hours

The fibromyalgia (FM) definition, according to the CDC via the American College of Rheumatology (ACR) in 1990, is a history of widespread pain. The patient must be experiencing pain or achiness, steady or intermittent, for at least three months. At times, the pain must have been present:

- On both sides of the body
- Both above and below the waist
- Mid-body. For example, in the neck, mid-chest, mid-back, or headache.
- Pain on at least eleven of the eighteen tender points

These current standards and definitions are not without flaws, such as requiring that the individual must have experienced six consecutive months of fatigue, which does not allow for the waxing and waning nature of the disease. They also require the individual to meet four minor criteria, and the diagnosis is dismissed when those aren't met, even if the individual has other symptoms associated with the condition. Also, the diagnosis is excluded if the individual has other known fatiguing conditions; however, the unique physiological hallmarks of CFS and FM don't exist in other fatiguing illnesses.

The above definitions for CFS and FM are strictly research definitions, and they exclude the majority of people who suffer from these syndromes. Since they also fail to address the underlying causes of the diseases, physicians are left without incentive to determine the underlying abnormalities, leading to treatments that are limited to simple symptomatic therapies.

Instead of defaulting to these standards, the quickest way to diagnose these conditions is by using the following definition: unexplained fatigue that significantly interferes with functioning and is associated with any *two* of the following:

- Brain fog
- Unrestful sleep
- Diffuse achiness
- Bowel dysfunction
- Unexplained neuropathy
- Recurrent and/or persistent infections or flu-like symptoms
- Postexertional malaise

It is important to remember when diagnosing these conditions that there are overlapping syndromes associated with CFS and FM, including: chronic fatigue immune dysfunction syndrome (CFIDS), myalgic encephalomyelitis (ME), multiple chemical sensitivity (MCS), chronic Lyme disease, chronic babesiosis, and Gulf War syndrome (GWS). All of these have the same underlying pathophysiology and, unfortunately, are poorly treated in the "standard medical care" given in the United States.

If the CDC criteria are met, the diagnosis of CFS carries a high specificity (very few false positives) and is associated with numerous documented physiological abnormalities with a specificity that is not obtained with many other diseases. For example, it has been shown that in patients diagnosed with both lupus and FM, it is more likely that the individual has FM and that lupus is a misdiagnosis. Although it is possible to have both conditions, the underlying pathophysiology is usually more consistent with FM, which means the appropriate treatment would be for FM and not lupus.

Studies suggest that 11.9% of the population currently experiences "severe fatigue, extreme tiredness or exhaustion" lasting over one month. Twenty-five to fifty percent of the general population complains of fatigue.

Twenty-five to forty percent of patients in a primary care setting complain of chronic fatigue and 4.2% have had these symptoms for over six months. An epidemiological study conducted in Australia investigated the impact of CFS on patients' lives and found that 43% of patients who met the criteria for CFS were disabled to such a degree that they were unable to attend school or work. A large study published in 1996 found that the degree of disability for people with CFS was greater than those with hypertension, congestive heart failure, type II diabetes mellitus, acute myocardial infarction, multiple sclerosis, and depression.[4] A Danish study demonstrated that CFS is more disabling than just about every other major illness.[5]

Problems with Standard Treatment of CFS and FM

Unfortunately, when it comes to treating patients with CFS and FM, doctors are often at a loss because either they can't figure out what's wrong (dismissing CFS/FM as "wastebasket" diagnoses) or they simply dismiss the symptoms as psychiatric in nature. As a result, fewer than 10%–30% of CFS patients have been given a correct diagnosis. Furthermore, the standard medical care for CFS and FM patients, which includes muscle relaxants, antidepressants, NSAIDs, passive stretching, and graded exercise, only minimally addresses the symptoms and ignores the cause entirely.

If the treating physician continues on with standard medical care, the prognosis of CFS is bleak. A five-year study concluded that "CFS patients exhibit severe, long-term function impairment." With standard care substantial improvement is very uncommon, less than 6%.[6] According to an American study, only 64% of patients reported a certain degree of improvement and only 2% experienced a complete recovery, with 40% remaining unable to work.[7]

A large multicenter study determined the long-term outcomes of FM in patients treated in rheumatology centers in which there was a special interest in the syndrome. Five hundred and thirty-eight patients being treated by rheumatologists who focus on FM, from six rheumatology centers, were assessed every six months for seven to ten years. The study found that functional disability worsened and measures of pain, global severity, fatigue, sleep disturbance, anxiety, depression, and health status were markedly abnormal at study initiation and were essentially unchanged over the study period. It concluded that "patients with established fibromyalgia, seen in rheumatology centers in which there is a special interest in the disease and followed up for as long as 7 years, have markedly abnormal scores for pain, functional disability, fatigue, sleep disturbance, and psychological status, and these values do not change substantially over time."[8]

A review published by Joyce and colleagues found that "after a review of 26 studies of the adults who met the CDC criteria of CFS had a poor prognosis with less than 10% recovering and the majority do not improve over time with standard medical care."[9]

Why are these conditions, CFS and FM, so poorly treated? There are a few reasons why patients with these debilitating conditions don't get the treatment and relief they need. First, only simple, symptomatic treatments are approved for FM, such as pregabalin, duloxetine, and milnacipran. Second, many doctors don't view these as real conditions. Their mindset is that if they cannot treat it, it must not be real. If they do acknowledge it, they don't know how to address it because of the poor knowledge base regarding pathophysiology and effective treatments of the conditions. A survey published in April 2005 found that approximately half of primary care physicians did not possess even a rudimentary knowledge of CFS or FM and were not confident in their ability to make either diagnosis.[10] Another survey published in 2005 also found that over half of the physicians did not possess enough knowledge to make the diagnosis, and even those who felt confident in making the diagnosis had a low level of specialist knowledge of these conditions. The authors concluded, "results from the study indicate that the level of specialist knowledge of CFS in primary care remains low . . . Steps are recommended to increase the knowledge base by compiling helpful and informative material for GPs . . ."[11] Third, standard laboratory tests are usually normal and there is no simple laboratory testing or simple treatment (multisystemic treatment is required for improvement). Fourth, health insurers can avoid paying for treatment and testing if they can make believe these syndromes are not real or physical. Fifth, 75% of those affected by these conditions are female. And finally, these conditions cannot be treated with the average fifteen-minute office visit.

Alternative Treatment of CFS and FM

While most physicians have the above-stated reservations, CFS and FM are very treatable conditions. When the multiple dysfunctions present are treated, significant improvement is seen, almost without exception. For instance, Teitelbaum and colleagues performed a randomized, double-blind, placebo-controlled, intent-to-treat study on 72 FM (69 also met CFS criteria) patients (38 active and 34 placebo) that documents the effectiveness of an integrative treatment approach to CFS and FM.[12] The patients underwent an integrative multisystem treatment protocol based on an algorithm that took into account laboratory tests as well as signs and symptoms. The study found that 57% of patients with CFS and/or FM had complete resolution of symptoms and 39% had incomplete but significant resolution of symptoms. A total of 96% had significant improvement or total resolution of symptoms.[13]

Our center tracked the treatment outcomes of over 500 consecutive CFS and FM patients. The results were peer-reviewed and published. The patients met the CDC criteria for CFS and/or the American College of Rheumatology criteria for FM (240 met criteria for CFS, 14 met criteria for FM, and 259 met criteria for both). The computerized system tracked each patient's average overall energy level and sense of well-being on each visit as well as the frequency and severity of ten symptoms, including fatigue, muscle pain, stiffness, cognitive function, headaches, insomnia, unrestful sleep, gastrointestinal dysfunction, and sore throat.[14]

Before each visit, patients rated their energy and sense of well-being on a scale of 1–10 (1 being low and 10 being high) and their individual symptom frequency and severity on a scale of 1–10 (10 being constant and 1 being rare for frequency, and 10 being severe and 1 being mild for severity). Patients had seen an average 7.2 different physicians for treatment of their CFS and/or FM without significant improvement prior to being seen at our center. Patients were treated based on a multisystem integrative treatment algorithm that incorporates therapies based on the most recent understanding of the pathophysiology of these conditions (due to its complexity, a description of the algorithm is beyond the scope of this chapter). The treatment algorithm included low dose naltrexone (LDN) if the symptoms or laboratory results were consistent with immune dysfunction. If patients met the protocol criteria, they were given a therapeutic trial of 4.5 mg of naltrexone at bedtime. Patients who reported "being sensitive" to medications were started on lower doses and titrated up as tolerated to 4.5–5.5 mg at bedtime. If patients complained of insomnia for more than two weeks, they were given the option to take the LDN during the day.[15]

Analysis revealed that 94% of patients had overall improvement by the fourth visit, with 75% noting significant overall improvement and 62%

reporting substantial overall improvement. The majority of patients continued to improve in subsequent visits. The average energy levels and average sense of well-being increased significantly.[16]

- 94% of patients had overall improvement by the fourth visit.
- 75% noted significant overall improvement.
- 62% reported substantial overall improvement.
- The average energy level and sense of well-being for patients doubled by the fourth visit.

Subsequently, over forty physicians were trained to utilize a more simplified treatment algorithm in seventeen centers across the country. In this multicenter study, over 4,000 consecutive patients diagnosed with CFS and/or FM were treated with this simplified algorithm that included LDN as a treatment option for those with immune dysfunction. The results were tracked via the same computerized patient assessment system. The data demonstrated that 85% of patients improved by the fourth visit, with 56% and 40% reporting significant and substantial improvement, respectively.[17]

In order to properly treat an individual with these conditions, the overall treatment can be grouped into different treatment phases:

- **Stabilize the patient.** Address the pain and sleep disturbances associated with these conditions with medication. However, the treating physician must remember that this is only the first step of many (most doctors don't treat beyond this step).
- **Enhance mitochondrial function.** Mitochondrial dysfunction can help to explain the symptoms of CFS and FM. It is important to supply the mitochondria with the nutrients they require, including magnesium, carnitine, D-ribose, CoQ10, and glutathione.
- **Balance the hormones.** Peer-reviewed medical literature documents pituitary and hypothalamic dysfunction in patients with CFS and FM, which results in patients with multiple hormone deficiencies that must be addressed.[18]
- **Treat the immune dysfunction.** This phase may be the most important aspect of treatment. In our experience, if the immune system is not addressed (maybe only one or two other phases are utilized), then long-term success is unlikely. The therapeutic trial of LDN should be considered in the majority of these patients not

on narcotic pain medication. Other options include medications such as Leukine or Neupogen, ozone via indirect IV (major autoheme); direct IV, intravenous ozonated saline, HOCATT, or rectal insufflation; isoprinosine, pulsed electromagnetic field therapy; gamma globulin; biomodulation; cryotherapy; Medsonix, low-dose immunotherapy, low-dose allergen, and a number of immune modulating herbal products such as mushroom extracts, Immunostim, and Cytoquel, to name a few.

- **Treat the infectious/immune components.** Medical literature documents the multiple infections that may either cause or contribute to CFS and FM, including Lyme disease and other strains of *Borrelia*, *Babesia*, *Bartonella*, Q-fever, *Mycoplasma*, human herpesvirus 6 (HHV6), Epstein-Barr virus (EBV), toxic mold, and *Candida*.[19]
- **Address unique etiologies.** This includes heavy metal toxicity, leaky gut (food allergies), toxic molds, and abnormal immune activation of coagulation (studies have found that 60%–90% of CFS, FM, and GWS patients have abnormal activation of the clotting system).
- **Adjust treatment as needed.** Adjustment of therapies will need to take place over time to wean the patient to the minimal core treatments. This can happen as improvements occur and the individual can discontinue certain medications.

While they are all important, the two components requiring special attention are the fourth and fifth: treat the infectious and immune components. This can be done through an evaluation for organisms through a history and physical, questionnaire, and testing for bacterial and viral infections as well as parasites and yeast. Next, the organisms may need to be eradicated through antibiotics, antivirals, or antifungals, and IV/PO (intravenous or oral) nutritional supplementation. However, the newest clinical experience shows that direct treatment of the invading organism may not be necessary or beneficial if the immune dysfunction is addressed.

Patients with CFS or FM have a TH1 (T-helper 1) to TH2 (T-helper 2) imbalance. TH1 helps the immune system fight against intracellular pathogens such as viruses, yeast, and some bacteria. TH2 helps the immune system fight extracellular pathogens such as parasites, allergens, and other toxins.

CFS and FM result in an individual being "stuck" in a TH2-dominant state. This means that immune-modulatory treatment is key to the successful treatment of chronic infections and CFS or FM. The best laboratory markers to determine whether the patient has an immune dysfunction that is the cause or a contributor of the illness is a low natural killer (NK) cell function (less than 30); a low CD 57 level; elevated C4a, high or low vascular endothelial growth factor (VEGF), high eosinophil cationic protein (ECP), angiotensin converting enzyme (ACE) above 30; or immune activation of coagulation (elevated d-dimer, prothrombin-antithrobin level, prothrombin fragment 1&2, soluble fibrin monomer, or PAI-1); or abnormal immunoglobulins or immunoglobulin G (IgG) subclass. The immune dysfunction allows opportunistic organisms and other infections to flourish, which amplifies the dysfunction. The infections can include a variety of infectious forms discussed above. While various antimicrobial treatments directed at such infections can certainly be beneficial, unless the immune system's inability to clear the infections is addressed, long-term success is unlikely. Although this is a gross oversimplification, the goal of immune modulation is to increase TH1 immunity and to decrease the TH2. There are major exceptions to this rule, but it can be used as a general model. This also means that the NK cell function needs to be increased while lowering inflammatory cytokines.

LDN underwent a pilot study on 12 FM patients, with a placebo-controlled, single-blind, crossover design. The study involved daily self-reported symptoms: baseline (two weeks), placebo (two weeks), and LDN (eight weeks). The primary outcome of self-reported overall FM symptom severity, secondary symptoms severity, and mechanical pain testing showed that LDN reduced FM symptoms by 30%.[20]

Another study reported similar results. This study was conducted on 32 FM patients, and also had a randomized, double-blind, placebo-controlled, crossover design. The study involved daily self-reported symptoms: baseline (two weeks), placebo (four weeks), or LDN (twelve weeks) and four-week follow-up. The primary outcome of self-reported overall FM severity, secondary symptom severity, and mechanical pain testing showed that LDN reduced FM symptoms by 28.8% versus 18% with placebo. LDN was also associated with improved mood and improved satisfaction with life. Thirty-two percent of the individuals met the criteria for response, which was defined as a significant reduction in pain, as well as a significant reduction in either fatigue or sleeplessness.[21]

Conclusion

Our centers have specialized in the treatment of CFS and FM for the past fifteen years. Rarely does a day go by when I don't see someone who has been devastated by these illnesses. It is heartbreaking that the overwhelming majority of physicians lack the tools, knowledge, and even the interest to effectively treat such patients. The "modern" medical system in this country has created huge roadblocks and disincentives for doctors to effectively treat these complex illnesses, so they must rely on simple FDA-approved medications that don't address the underlying abnormalities, and are frankly not much better than placebo. In fact, they often prove to be worse than placebo because of the risks of side effects. This complaint has been echoed by the majority of doctors who specialize in the treatment of CFS and FM.

This raises the question as to how these ineffective medications got approved as standard-of-care treatments in the first place. While the answer is complex and multifactorial, one major reason is patient selection. All of the study designs have thus far been on patients with mild to moderate cases who are on no medications or treatments and have no other diagnosed comorbidities (comorbidity is a hallmark of these illnesses), because other medications and comorbidities may confound the results. While it can be argued that this is necessary to simplify the study design, such a group represents only a small percentage of patients seen by physicians; only a small percentage of patients fit such criteria. Most patients with CFS and FM have a very complex set of symptoms with multiple prior diagnoses, and have tried numerous therapies without success. These patients almost always have multiple comorbidities, which are considered unrelated to the illness, therefore disqualifying them from the study trial. However, when the illness is properly and comprehensively treated, these so-called unrelated comorbidities go away.

Having treated patients with CFS and FM for the past fifteen years, I have come to the conclusion that I cannot do so effectively if I am forced to see them for fifteen minutes or less each visit. A visit must be comprehensive and usually requires an hour to adequately assess the progress of the patient, rather than the standard ten- to twenty-minute visit that is reimbursed by insurance companies and paid for by a patient's co-pay. Since most medical practices are insurance-based businesses, doctors can only afford to spend fifteen minutes per patient. A complete overhaul of medical business practice would have to be undertaken in order to see fewer numbers of these complex patients per day, since the current system rewards high patient volume. Doctors are forced to choose between high patient volume with superficial, ineffective care in order to pay the bills, and comprehensive care with a dramatically lower patient volume that isn't economically feasible. In addition to the financial constraints, there is increased paperwork, increased interaction with insurance companies and pharmacies for prior authorization of unapproved medication, and increased scrutiny by medical boards due to the "alternative" approach. This is simply a fact of the current state of the American health care system.

Every doctor who treats the general public faces the same philosophical dilemma: continue rushing through patient visits and writing out prescriptions for medications that are ineffective at best, and often harmful to the patient, or seek a different path. Unfortunately, until the current medical system is redesigned, the only other path available to doctors with integrity and passion appears to be to opt out of insurance-based practices and take the risk of running a cash-based practice, requiring considerable risk as well as the need to raise fees, which prices out a huge percentage of their patients. This is the situation we now find ourselves in.

Why do I emphasize this current predicament in a book about LDN? Because LDN has proven so effective that doctors can prescribe it with reasonable hope that patients will improve without extensive time and multiple interventions. While nothing works for everyone, LDN has some benefit in most patients and has a dramatic effect in a good percentage. The key is that there are no significant side effects. Only a small percentage of patients report minor side effects, and I have never seen a major side effect, unless given concurrently with a contraindicated opioid drug. This allows doctors who care about their patients to stay within "the system" until another alternative proves feasible.

FIVE

Thyroid Disorders

KENT HOLTORF, MD

Low dose naltrexone (LDN) has been shown to be very effective in the treatment of autoimmune thyroiditis, including Graves' disease and Hashimoto's disease. Both conditions are caused by an unbalanced immune system where the immune system attacks the thyroid as if it were an invading organism. In the case of Graves' disease, the antibodies stimulate the thyroid receptor, resulting in hyperthyroidism (too much thyroid hormone produced). In the case of Hashimoto's disease, the antibodies and subsequent inflammation slowly destroy the thyroid gland tissue, resulting in hypothyroidism (too little thyroid hormone produced). LDN is shown to modulate the immune system and reduce the abnormal production of antibodies causing these disorders.

Patients and most doctors, including endocrinologists, are taught that Hashimoto's disease is the most common cause of hypothyroidism, but the incidence of Hashimoto's disease is only a fraction of those who suffer from low cellular thyroid levels. The difference is that Hashimoto's disease is generally easy to diagnose, while the large percentage of the population who suffer from cellular hypothyroidism almost always go undiagnosed because standard thyroid testing, including measurements of thyroid-stimulating hormone (TSH), free T3, and free T4, fails to detect such dysfunction the majority of the time.

Most, if not all, patients who suffer from depression, obesity, diabetes, insulin resistance, premenstrual syndrome (PMS), chronic dieting, stress, chronic fatigue syndrome, and fibromyalgia have immune dysfunction that results in low tissue levels of thyroid hormone. The immune dysfunction and inflammation causes hypothalamic and pituitary dysfunction (reduced secretion of TSH), reduced conversion of T4 to T3, increased T4 to reverse

T3 conversion, reduced thyroid hormone transport into the cell, and thyroid resistance (the same amount of thyroid in the blood has less of response). Unfortunately, standard thyroid function tests do not detect these more common causes of tissue hypothyroidism.

There have been exciting advances in the understanding of the local control of thyroid metabolism, including deiodinase activity and thyroid hormone membrane transport. The goal of this chapter is to increase the understanding of the clinical relevance of cellular deiodinase activity. The physiological significance of types 1, 2, and 3 deiodinase (D1, D2, and D3, respectively) on the intracellular production of T3 are discussed, along with the importance and significance of the production of reverse T3. The difference in the pituitary and peripheral activity of these deiodinases under a wide range of common physiological conditions results in desperate intracellular T3 levels in the pituitary and peripheral tissues, resulting in the inability to detect low tissue levels of thyroid hormone in peripheral tissues with TSH testing.

This chapter demonstrates that extreme caution should be used in relying on TSH or serum thyroid levels to rule out hypothyroidism in the presence of a wide range of conditions, including physiological and emotional stress, depression, dieting, obesity, leptin insulin resistance, diabetes, chronic fatigue syndrome, fibromyalgia, inflammation, autoimmune diseases, and systemic illnesses, as TSH levels will often be normal despite the presence of significant hypothyroidism. The chapter discusses the significant clinical benefit of thyroid replacement in such conditions despite having normal TSH levels, and the superiority of T3 instead of standard T4 therapy. The unique ability of LDN to modulate the immune system, cytokine production, and chronic inflammation can potentially improve the abnormal inflammation and immune dysfunction, and thus, improve the reduced tissue T3 levels seen with the above conditions. Consequentially, LDN can, by improving tissue thyroid levels, be very effective in the treatment of thyroid dysfunction seen with the majority of chronic illnesses.

Autoimmune Thyroiditis

Mounting evidence is demonstrating that LDN is an effective treatment for a wide range of autoimmune diseases, including Hashimoto's disease and Graves' disease. Hashimoto's is diagnosed by the presence of a significant amount of serum antibodies that attack the thyroid, including antithyroglobulin antibody and antithyroid peroxidase (anti-TPO) antibody. These antibodies progressively damage the thyroid, resulting in primary hypothyroidism due to decreased thyroid hormone production by the thyroid gland. If there is an antithyroid antibody that attaches to the TSH receptor, the thyroid is stimulated, resulting in hyperthyroidism. Such abnormalities are not usually checked by most doctors, and endocrinologists feel there is no effective treatment, which is proving to be untrue. There are some minerals, such as selenium and herbal treatments, that can slightly reduce the production of autoantibodies that cause Hashimoto's disease and Graves' disease. However, the immunomodulatory effects of LDN are showing significant promise in reducing the production of autoantibodies in a wide range of diseases, including Hashimoto's disease and Graves' disease, and are emerging as the first line in the treatment of these conditions.

Deiodinase Enzymes

To accurately assess thyroid function, it must be understood that deiodinase enzymes are essential control points of cellular thyroid activity that determine intracellular activation and deactivation of thyroid hormones. This local control of cellular thyroid levels is mediated through three different deiodinase enzymes present in different tissues in the body; type I deiodinase (D1) and type II deiodinase (D2) increase cellular thyroid activity by converting inactive thyroxine (T4) to the active triiodothyronine (T3), while type III deiodinase (D3) reduces cellular thyroid activity by converting T4 to the antithyroid reverse T3 (reverse T3).[1]

The activity of each type of deiodinase enzyme changes in response to differing physiological conditions, and this local control of intracellular T4 and T3 levels results in different tissue levels of T4 and T3 under different conditions. Because it is the activity of these deiodinases and transport of T4 and T3 into the cell that determine tissue and cellular thyroid levels and not serum thyroid levels, serum thyroid hormone levels may not necessarily predict tissue thyroid levels under a variety of physiological conditions.

DEIODINASE TYPE 1 (D1)

D1 converts inactive T4 to active T3 throughout the body, but D1 is not a significant determinant of pituitary T4 to T3 conversion, which is controlled by D2.[2] D1 but not D2 is suppressed and down-regulated (decreasing T4 to T3 conversion) in response to physiological and emotional stress;[3] depression;[4] dieting;[5] weight gain and leptin resistance;[6] insulin resistance, obesity, and diabetes;[7] inflammation from autoimmune diseases or systemic illnesses;[8] chronic fatigue syndrome and fibromyalgia;[9] chronic pain;[10] and exposure to toxins and plastics.[11] In the presence of such conditions there are reduced tissue levels of active thyroid in all tissues except the pituitary. The reduced thyroid tissue levels with these conditions is often quoted as a beneficial response that lowers metabolism and thus does not require treatment, but there is no evidence to support such a stance, while there is significant evidence demonstrating that it is a detrimental response.[12]

In addition, D1 activity is also lower in females,[13] making women more prone to tissue hypothyroidism, with resultant depression, fatigue, fibromyalgia, chronic fatigue syndrome, and obesity despite having normal TSH levels.

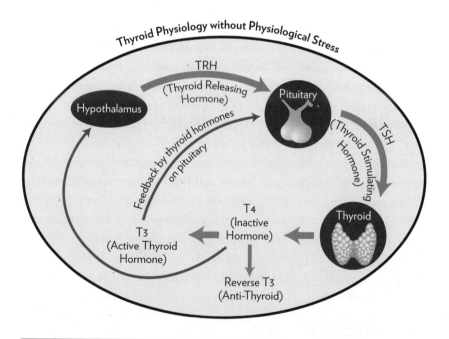

FIGURE 5.1. Peripheral thyroid hormone conversion and its impact on TSH and metabolic activity. Image by Kent Holtorf, MD

DEIODINASE TYPE II (D2)

Thyroid-stimulating hormone (TSH) is produced in the pituitary and is regulated by intrapituitary T3 levels, which often do not correlate or provide an accurate indicator of T3 levels in the rest of the body. Using the TSH as an indicator for the body's overall thyroid status assumes that the T3 levels in the pituitary directly correlate with that of other tissues in the body and that changes directly correlate with that of T3 in other tissues of the body under a wide range of physiological conditions. This, however, is shown not to be the case; the pituitary is different from every other tissue in the body.

Due to the unique makeup of deiodinases in the pituitary, it will respond differently and often opposite to that of every other tissue in the body. Numerous conditions result in an increase in pituitary T3 levels with a simultaneous suppression of cellular T3 levels in the rest of the body, making the pituitary, and thus the TSH, a poor indicator for tissue thyroid levels in the rest of the body under numerous physiological conditions.

In addition to having a unique makeup of deiodinases, the pituitary also contains unique membrane thyroid transporters and thyroid receptors. As opposed to the rest of the body that is regulated by both D1 and D3, the pituitary contains little D1 and no D3;[14] pituitary T3 levels are determined by D2 activity,[15] which is a thousand times more efficient at converting T4 to T3 than the D1 enzyme present in the rest of the body[16] and is much less sensitive to suppression by toxins and medications.[17] Though D2 activity is present in human skeletal muscle (unexpected from studies in rats), there is less D1 and D3 present in the pituitary than in the other tissues of the body.[18] In the pituitary, 80%–90% of T4 is converted to T3[19] while only about 30%–50% of T4 in the peripheral tissue is converted to active T3.[20] This is due to the inefficiency of D1 and the presence of D3 in all tissues of the body except the pituitary that competes with D1 and converts T4 to reverse T3.[21]

Additionally, D2 has an opposite response from that of D1 to physiological and emotional stress, depression, both dieting and weight gain, PMS, diabetes, leptin resistance, chronic fatigue syndrome, fibromyalgia, inflammation, autoimmune diseases, and systemic illnesses. D2 is stimulated and up-regulated (has increased activity) in response to such conditions, increasing intrapituitary T4 to T3 conversion, while the rest of body suffers from diminished levels of active T3. This causes the TSH to remain normal despite the fact that there is significant cellular hypothyroidism present in the rest of the body.

Thus, the pituitary levels are under completely different physiological control, and T3 levels will always be significantly higher than anywhere else in the body.[22] Consequently, if the TSH is elevated, even mildly, it is clear that many tissues of the body will be deficient in T3, but due to the different physiology, a normal TSH cannot be used as a reliable indicator for normal T3 levels in the rest of the body.

Different thyroid levels and conditions will have different effects on the T3 levels in the pituitary than in the rest of the body, resulting in different T3 levels in the pituitary and the rest of the body, making the TSH unreliable under numerous circumstances. For instance, as the levels of T4 decline, as in hypothyroidism, the activity of D2 increases and is able to partially compensate for the reduction in serum T4.[23] On the other hand, with reduced T4 levels, the activity and efficiency of D1 decreases[24] resulting in a reduction in cellular T3 levels, while the TSH remains unchanged due to the ability of the pituitary D2 to compensate for the diminished T4.

As stated above, this lack of correlation of TSH and peripheral tissue levels of T3 is dramatically worsened in numerous conditions. These include chronic emotional or physical stress, chronic illness, diabetes, insulin resistance, obesity, leptin resistance, depression, chronic fatigue syndrome, fibromyalgia, PMS, and both dieting and weight gain. In such conditions, tissue levels of T3 are shown to drop dramatically out of proportion with serum T3 levels.[25] While serum T3 levels may drop by 30%, which is significant but still may be in the so-called "normal" range, tissue T3 levels may drop by 70%–80%, resulting in profound cellular hypothyroidism with normal serum TSH, T4, and T3 levels.[26] Consequently, in the presence of such conditions, the TSH is a poor indicator for peripheral thyroid levels and a normal TSH should not be considered a reliable indicator for an individual being euthyroid (normal thyroid), especially in the presence of symptoms consistent with thyroid deficiency.

Lim and colleagues measured peripheral (liver) and pituitary levels of T3 in rats in response to induced chronic illness.[27] They found that pituitary T3 and TSH levels remained unchanged, while the peripheral tissues were significantly reduced. The authors summarized their findings by stating:

> *The reduction in hepatic nuclear T3 content and T3-Cmax in the Nx2 rats is consistent with the presence of selective tissue deficiency*

*of thyroid hormones. The pituitary, however, had normal T3
content, suggesting a dissociation in thyroid hormone-dependent
metabolic status between peripheral tissue (liver) and the pituitary. This explains the failure to observe an increase in serum
TSH level, a manifestation of reduced intracellular rather than
serum T3 concentration . . . Most interesting, we found that, in
contrast to the liver, the pituitary of the Nx rats was not deprived
of thyroid hormone. This finding offers a convincing explanation
of the failure to observe an increase of serum TSH when illness
or stress-induced reduction of hepatic T4 5'-monodeiodination
causes a fall in serum T3 concentration.[28]*

Larsen and colleagues summarized their finding that the pituitary has a
unique composition of deiodinases that is not present in any other tissue in
the body, making the pituitary T3 levels, and thus the TSH, a poor indicator
for tissue T3 in the rest of the body—stating that the TSH cannot be reliably
used as a marker of thyroid status in the rest of the body.[29]

*Changes in pituitary conversion of T4 to T3 are often opposite
of those that occur in the liver and kidney under similar circumstances. The presence of this pathway of T3 production indicates
that the pituitary can respond independently to changes in plasma
levels of T4 and T3 . . . Given these results, it is not surprising
that a complete definition of thyroid status requires more than the
measurement of the serum concentrations of thyroid hormones.
For some tissues, the intracellular T3 concentration may only
partially reflect those in the serum. Recognition that the intracellular T3 concentration in each tissue may be subject to local
regulation and an understanding of the importance of this process
to the regulation of TSH production should permit a better appre-
ciation of the limitations of the measurements of serum thyroid
hormone and TSH levels.[30]*

DEIODINASE TYPE III (D3)

The pituitary is the only tissue that does not contain D3,[31] which converts
T4 to reverse T3 and competes with D1 that converts T4 to T3.[32] Reverse

T3 is a competitive inhibitor of T3, blocking T3 from binding to its receptor and blocking T3 effect,[33] reducing metabolism,[34] suppressing D1 and T4 to T3 conversion,[35] and blocking T4 and T3 uptake into the cell,[36] all reducing intracellular T3 levels and thyroid activity. Because many tissues may have abundant D3 levels while the pituitary is uniquely void of D3,[37] the inhibitory effects on the peripheral tissues causing hypothyroidism are not reflected by TSH testing (see figures 5.1 and 5.3).

Reverse T3 is present in varying concentrations in different tissues and with different individuals.[38] It is up-regulated with chronic physiological stress and illness[39] and is an indicator for reduced T4 to T3 conversion and low intracellular T3 levels even if the TSH is normal.[40]

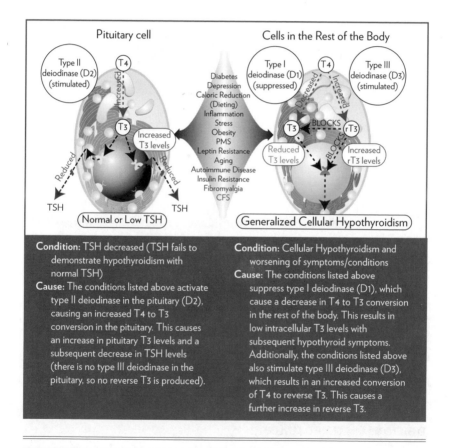

FIGURE 5.2. Conditions that cause low cellular T3 (hypothyroidism) not detected by TSH levels. Image by Kent Holtorf, MD

Because increased serum and tissue levels of reverse T3 will result in a blocking of the thyroid receptors, even small increases in reverse T3 can result in a significant decrease in thyroid action and result in severe hypothyroidism not detected by standard blood tests.[41] Because any T4 given will contribute to more reverse T3, T4-only preparations should not be considered optimal thyroid replacement in the presence of high or high-normal reverse T3 levels,[42] while T3 can be significantly beneficial.[43]

Pituitary Thyroid Transport and Deiodinase Activity Determines TSH Levels

The pituitary is different from every other cell in the body, with its own distinct deiodinases, thyroid transporters, and high-affinity thyroid receptors.[44] As mentioned previously, the pituitary thyroid hormone transporters are not energy dependent and can thus maintain or increase the cellular uptake of T4 and T3 even in low energy states.[45] This stands in stark contrast with transporters found in other parts of the body that would normally experience significantly reduced transport under similar circumstances.[46]

Stress

Chronic physiological stress results in decreased D1 activity[47] and an increase in D3 activity,[48] decreasing thyroid activity by converting T4 into reverse T3 instead of T3.[49] Conversely, D2 is stimulated, which results in increased T4 to T3 conversion in the pituitary and reduced production of TSH.[50] The increased cortisol levels seen with stress also contribute to a physiological disconnect between the TSH and peripheral tissue T3 levels.[51] This stress-induced reduced tissue T3 level and increased reverse T3 results in tissue hypothyroidism and potential weight gain, fatigue, and depression.[52] The vicious cycle of weight gain, fatigue, and depression that is associated with stress can be prevented with supplementation with timed-released T3[53] but not T4.[54]

Chronic emotional or physiological stress can cause significant reduction of transport of T4 into the cells of the body. For example, Sarne and colleagues added serum from different groups of individuals to cell cultures and measured the amount of T4 uptake from the serum into the cell. Their results showed that the serum from those with significant physiological stress inhibited the uptake (transport) of T4 into the cell while the serum from the nonphysiologically stressed had no effect.[55] These results demonstrate that

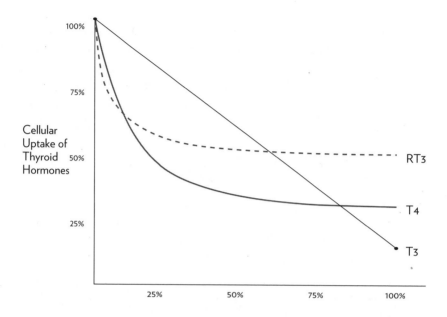

Percent drop in cellular energy (above) and severity of stress, depression, cholesterol level, insulin resistance, and dieting (below)

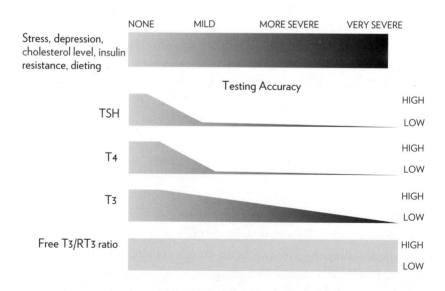

FIGURE 5.3. Thyroid hormone transport into cellular tissue.

serum T4 levels can be artificially elevated among physiologically stressed individuals and, thus, serum T4 and TSH levels are poor markers for tissue thyroid levels in this patient population (see figure 5.2).[56] Substances produced by physiological stress or calorie reduction (e.g., 3-carboxy-4-methyl-5-propyl-2-furan propanoic acid [CMPF], indoxyl sulfate, bilirubin, and fatty acids) have been shown to reduce the cellular uptake of T4 by up to 42%, while having no effect on T4 or T3 uptake into the pituitary.[57]

In addition to the above, numerous other studies have linked physiological stress to reduced cellular uptake of T4 and T3. For instance, Arem and colleagues found that significant physiological stress was associated with dramatically reduced tissue levels of T4 and T3 (up to 79%) without a corresponding increase in TSH.[58] The authors also found there was tissue variability in the level of suppression in different tissues, resulting in a significant variation when comparing the T4 and T3 levels in different tissues. This large variation of T4 and T3 levels in different tissues may explain the wide range and variation in individual symptoms of hypothyroidism.[59]

The reduced immunity from chronic stress has been thought to be due to excess cortisol production, but the associated reduction in tissue thyroid levels is shown to play a larger role in the decreased immunity seen with stress, and thyroid supplementation is shown to reverse the stress-induced reduction in immunity.[60]

As with stress, treatment with prednisone or other glucocorticoid will suppress D1 and stimulate D3, reducing T4 to T3 conversion and increasing T4 to reverse T3, causing a relative tissue hypothyroidism that is not detected by TSH testing.[61] This low cellular thyroid level certainly contributes to the weight gain and other associated side effects with such treatment. Thus, in stressed patients or those treated with corticosteroids, there are reduced tissue T3 levels that are not reflected by the TSH level, making the TSH an inappropriate marker for tissue levels of T3.

Depression

Many depressed and bipolar patients have undiagnosed thyroid dysfunction as the underlying cause or major contributor to their depression.[62] The dysfunction present with these conditions includes down-regulation of D1 (reduced T4 to T3 conversion) and reduced uptake of T4 into the cell, resulting in increased serum T4 levels with low intracellular T3 levels and up-regulated

D3, resulting in elevated reverse T3,[63] which blocks the thyroid effect[64] and is an indicator of reduced transport of T4 into the cell.[65] Additionally, studies show that depressed patients have reduced T4 transport across the blood brain barrier due to a defective transport protein, transthyretin, resulting in significantly reduced thyroid levels in the brains of depressed patients despite "normal" serum levels and standard thyroid tests[66] as well as a reduced TSH response to thyroid-releasing hormone (TRH).[67]

It is not surprising that T4 and T4/T3 combinations may have some benefit in depression, but due to the suppressed T4 to T3 conversion from suppressed D1and reduced uptake of T4 into the cell and brain,[68] timed-released T3 is significantly more beneficial than T4 or T4/T3 combination supplementation.[69]

Posternak and colleagues held a double-blind placebo-controlled trial of 50 patients with normal thyroid function as defined by a normal TSH (1.5+/- 0.8). The patients were randomized to receive 25 micrograms (µg) of T3 or placebo in addition to antidepressant therapy.[70] The study found an almost twofold increase in response rate with T3 and a 4.5 times greater likelihood of experiencing a positive response at any point over a six-week period with the addition of T3. Side effects were higher in the placebo group on ten of eleven criteria, including a significant increase in nervousness.

Kelly and colleagues investigated the effectiveness of T3 for the treatment of bipolar disorder in patients who had failed to adequately respond to an average of fourteen medications used to treat their bipolar disorder. The average dose of T3 used was 90.4 µg (from a range of 13–188 µg). The medication was found to be well tolerated, and 84% experienced significant improvement, with 33% having a full remission. Again, this is in patients who had not previously responded to numerous medications. One patient who was switched to T4 for cost reasons experienced a return of symptoms, which resolved with the reintroduction of T3. The authors concluded, "Augmentation with supraphysiological doses of T3 should be considered in cases of treatment resistant bipolar depression."[71] The authors thanked several doctors who encouraged them to go beyond the traditional 50 µg of T3 because it has helped so many of their patients.

With over 4,000 patients, the Star*D Report is the largest trial comparing antidepressant effectiveness for depression. It found that 66% of patients failed to respond to antidepressants or had side effects severe enough to discontinue use. Of those who did respond, over half relapsed within one year.[72] The trial found that T3 was effective even when other medications such as citalopram (Celexa), bupropion (Wellbutrin), sertraline (Zoloft), venlafaxine (Effexor), or cognitive therapy were not. T3 was shown to be 50% more effective, even with the less-than-optimal dose of 50 μg, under direct comparison, with significantly less side effects than commonly used therapeutic approaches with standard antidepressants. The authors included a case study to exemplify the effectiveness of T3, especially when other medications are not:

> Ms. "B," a 44-year-old divorced white woman, became depressed after losing her job as a secretary in a law firm. She initially sought treatment from her primary care physician and then entered the STAR*D study. Ms. B met criteria for major depressive disorder and generalized anxiety disorder. Her baseline QIDS-SR score was 16. After 12 weeks on citalopram, her QIDS-SR score was 10 [minimal response]. She was then randomly assigned to augmentation with buspirone; she soon experienced gastrointestinal distress, and she stopped taking buspirone after 6 weeks. She elected to try one more augmentation agent and was randomly assigned to T3 augmentation. When she started T3 augmentation, her QIDS-SR score was 12. After 4 weeks, she felt that her mood and energy had lifted substantially. She felt better able to make decisions, organize, and prioritize and felt that she was able and ready to look for another job. "I felt as if my brain suddenly had oxygen," she said, "and everything became clearer." After 12 weeks, Ms. B felt back to normal, and her QIDS-SR score was 0.[73]

With an understanding of thyroid physiology and the associated dysfunction that is present in depressed patients, it is clear that timed-released T3 supplementation should be considered in all depressed and bipolar patients despite "normal" serum thyroid levels. Additionally, straight T4 should be considered inappropriate and suboptimal therapy for replacement in such patients.

Pain

Chronic pain will significantly suppress D1 and up-regulate D2, resulting in a reduction in tissue T3 without a change in TSH.[74] Thus, significant cellular hypothyroidism is not detected by serum TSH and T4 testing.[75] This cellular hypothyroidism, which again is undiagnosed by standard blood tests, increases the risk of the associated fatigue and depression seen with chronic pain.[76]

Narcotic pain medication can, of course, alleviate pain and thus potentially improve the diminished tissue T3 levels seen with chronic pain, but narcotics also suppress D1 but not D2, so such treatment is also a cause of low tissue levels of T3 accompanied by a normal TSH, and so again the tissue hypothyroidism remains undetected.[77]

Exercise

It has been shown that women or men who perform more than moderate exercise, especially when associated with dieting, have reduced T4 to T3 conversion and increase reverse T3, counteracting many of the positive effects of exercise, including weight loss.[78] Consequently, T3 and reverse T3 levels should be evaluated in individuals who exercise and/or diet to better determine cellular thyroid levels, as TSH and T4 would not necessarily reflect tissue levels in such patients.

Dieting

In a highly controlled study, Brownell and colleagues found that after repeated cycles of dieting, weight loss occurred at half the rate and weight gain occurred at three times the rate compared to controls with the same calorie intake.[79] Furthermore, severe caloric restriction and weight cycling is shown to be associated with reduced cellular T4 uptake of 25%–50%.[80] Therefore, successful weight loss is doomed to failure unless the reduced intracellular thyroid levels are addressed, but, as stated previously, this reduced cellular thyroid level is generally not detected by standard laboratory testing. Van der Heyden and colleagues studied the effect of calorie restriction (dieting) on the transport of T4 and T3 into the cell.[81] They found that obese individuals in the processes of dieting exhibited a 50% reduction of T4 into the cell and a 25% reduction of T3 into the cell. This is thought to be due to the reduced cellular energy stores as well as increased levels of free fatty acids and nonesterified fatty acids in the serum. This data helps explain why standard thyroid blood tests are not accurate indicators of intracellular thyroid levels. It also explains why it is difficult for obese patients to lose weight: as calories are decreased, thyroid utilization is reduced and metabolism drops. Among patients with this type of thyroid hormone transport dysfunction (resulting in intracellular hypothyroidism), assessing the free T3 to reverse T3 ratio can aid in a proper diagnosis, with a free T3 to reverse T3 ratio of less than 0.2 being a marker for tissue hypothyroidism (when the free T3 is expressed in picograms per milliliter [2.3–4.2 pg/mL] and the reverse T3 is expressed in nanograms per deciliter [8–25 ng/dL]) (see figure 5.2).[82]

Iron Deficiency

Iron deficiency is shown to significantly reduce T4 to T3 conversion, increase reverse T3 levels, and block the thermogenic (metabolism boosting) properties of thyroid hormone.[83] Thus, iron deficiency, as indicated by an iron saturation below 25 or a ferritin below 70, will result in diminished intracellular T3 levels. Additionally, T4 should not be considered adequate thyroid replacement if iron deficiency is present due to the lack of T4 to T3 conversion.[84]

Inflammation Associated with Common Conditions

The inflammatory cytokines IL-1, Il-6, C-reactive protein, and TNF-α will significantly decrease D1 activity and reduce tissue T3 levels.[85] Any person with an inflammatory condition—including physical or emotional stress,[86] obesity,[87] diabetes,[88] depression,[89] menopause (surgical or natural),[90] heart disease,[91] autoimmune diseases (lupus, Hashimoto's disease, multiple sclerosis, arthritis, etc.),[92] injury,[93] chronic infection,[94] or cancer[95]—will have a decreased T4 to T3 conversion in the body and a relative tissue hypothyroidism. The inflammatory cytokines will, however, increase the activity of D2 and suppress the TSH despite reduced peripheral T3 levels, again, making a normal TSH an unreliable indicator of normal tissue thyroid levels.

Individual Variations in Deiodinase Activity

The relative amounts of D1, D2, and D3 vary in different tissues among different individuals[96] and under varying conditions,[97] resulting in hundreds of possible symptoms with hypothyroidism; some people have one symptom, some have a few, and some people have many, depending on the relative level of T3 in each tissue. Unfortunately, serum thyroid levels often do not accurately reflect intracellular tissue levels or levels in a particular tissue.

LDN and Thyroid Utilization

A large number of studies are proving that LDN can effectively reduce abnormal inflammation and cytokine production and effectively normalize immune abnormalities. As expected as a result of such effects, LDN is showing ability to improve the transport of thyroid hormones into the cells, increase T4 to T3 conversion and reduce T4 to reverse T3 conversion. Thus, LDN can reverse the causes of the thyroid resistance that are shown to be present in the majority of people in the United States and the world. As expected, LDN can be beneficial in the treatment of not only autoimmune diseases, but also depression, insulin resistance, diabetes, obesity, anxiety, neurodegenerative diseases, chronic fatigue syndrome, fibromyalgia, hypercholesterolemia, and other chronic illnesses. The increased thyroid utilization also makes it beneficial for weight loss (it is an FDA-approved component for weight loss).

EXAMPLE OF CLINICAL EFFECTS OF LDN

We see many patients with elevated TPO and antithyroglobulin antibodies (Hashimoto's disease) and thyroid-stimulating immunoglobulin (TSI) antibodies (Graves' disease) that are successfully treated with LDN. While LDN does not work for everyone, a large percentage of patients will see a significant reduction in autoantibodies when treated with LDN.

We also see many patients, especially women, who complain of a wide array of symptoms commonly seen with hypothyroidism, such as fatigue, inability to lose weight, cold hands and feet, cold intolerance, irregular periods, PMS, dry and brittle hair, or diffuse hair loss on scalp, but have seemingly normal serum thyroid levels. They often have a low-normal TSH and high-normal free T4, a low-normal free T3, a high-normal reverse T3, and a sex hormone-binding globulin (SHBG) below 60 nmol/L, which are markers of thyroid resistance (diminished conversion of T4 to T3 and reduced cellular thyroid transport into cells). They usually have a slow relaxation phase of the brachioradialis reflex (RBR)—slower than 110 milliseconds—and low resting metabolic rates (RMR).

After treatment with LDN, patients often see significant improvement in their symptoms and improved RBR and RMR, all being consistent with improved utilization of thyroid hormone at the cellular level, which is likely due to increased thyroid hormone transport into the peripheral tissue and increased conversion of T4 to T3 (and reduced T4 to reverse T3). Their free

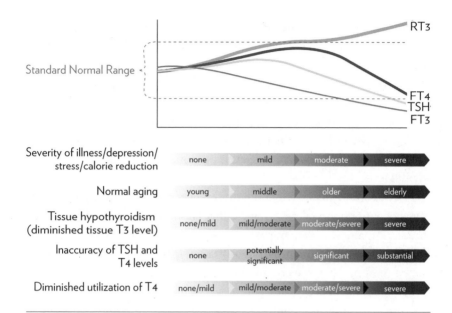

FIGURE 5.4. Associated serum thyroid levels with progressively decreasing tissue thyroid levels due to stress, illness, depression, calorie reduction, or aging (why standard blood tests lack sensitivity to detect low thyroid in the presence of such conditions). Demonstrates why TSH levels lack the accuracy to detect cellular levels and the free T3/reverseT3 ratio is the most accurate method to determine cellular thyroid levels in the presence of physiologic stress, depression, or obesity. Image by Kent Holtorf, MD

T4 decreases, showing improved transport of T4 into the cell and increased conversion to T3;[98] their TSH usually increases slightly, showing a reduction of inflammation-induced suppression of TSH; their free T3 levels either decrease slightly or remain unchanged, showing increased transport of T3 into the cell but not as much decrease as T4 because the increased transport is partially compensated for by the increased T4 to T3 conversion; their reverse T3 declines significantly, showing reduced conversion of T4 to reverse T3, also indicating increased transport of T4 into the cell, and their SHBG increases, demonstrating improved cellular thyroid levels.[99]

Summary

With an improved understanding of thyroid physiology that includes the local control of intracellular activation and deactivation of thyroid hormones by deiodinases, it becomes clear that standard thyroid tests often do not reflect the thyroid status in the tissues of the body other than the pituitary. This is especially true with physiological and emotional stress, depression, dieting, obesity, leptin insulin resistance, diabetes, chronic fatigue syndrome and fibromyalgia, inflammation, autoimmune diseases, and systemic illnesses. Consequently, it is inappropriate to rely on a normal TSH, free T4, or free T3 as adequate or sensitive indicators of normal or low tissue levels of T3 in the presence of any such conditions, making the TSH and other thyroid hormone levels poor markers for the body's overall thyroid level.

LDN is shown to improve the underlying pathophysiology of a wide range of autoimmune illnesses, including Hashimoto's disease and Graves' disease. It is also shown to improve the underdiagnosed but common problem of diminished cellular thyroid utilization (thyroid resistance), which is shown to occur with the common conditions listed above. Having a very low risk and incidence of side effects, a trial of LDN should be considered with any patient having symptoms suggestive of hypothyroidism or any of the common diseases listed above.

SIX

Restless Legs Syndrome

Leonard B. Weinstock, MD, FACG, and Trisha L. Myers, PA-CMD

There are three basic categories of restless legs syndrome (RLS), which has recently been renamed Willis-Ekbom disease: idiopathic primary RLS, familial RLS, and secondary RLS. In all categories of this commonly occurring syndrome, four primary symptoms are present: (1) the compelling urge to move the extremities, usually the legs, often associated with discomfort; (2) occurrence during rest or inactivity; (3) occurrence or worsening typically in the evening; and (4) temporary improvement with movement, including stretching or walking. With respect to secondary RLS, over fifty diseases, disorders, and conditions have been reported to be associated with and/or contribute to RLS.[1] In a recent publication we reviewed all of these disorders and conditions and found that most have the potential to cause systemic inflammation and/or immune disorders. Idiopathic RLS has been shown to be associated with small intestinal bacterial overgrowth (SIBO), and preliminary evidence suggests that treating the underlying gastrointestinal disorder can improve RLS severity. Clinical experience suggests that treatment against inflammation per se may be beneficial in RLS.

In this chapter, RLS is reviewed and its pathophysiology is discussed. Central nervous system (CNS) endorphin deficiency, altered dopamine interactions, and central iron deficiency due to inflammation are discussed as RLS pathophysiology for which LDN may play a role in therapy. Preliminary experience with LDN in RLS patients with and without SIBO will be reviewed.

History and Definition of RLS

Restless legs syndrome is a CNS disorder that is either idiopathic or secondary to a number of conditions. Some cases of RLS may, however, be directly related to peripheral neuropathy. The primary symptom of RLS is the compelling urge to move the legs at night, often with discomfort. The prevalence is estimated at 5%–10% of the general population, and it results in sleep disorders and poor quality of life.[2]

Restless legs syndrome was first described in the English literature by Thomas Willis in 1695 as "restlessness . . . as if they were in a place of greatest torture." He treated the condition with a narcotic (laudanum), which relates to recent opioid and LDN treatment of RLS. In 1945 a treatise by Karl-Axel Ekbom further defined the syndrome. In part due to recognition of these individuals, the Restless Legs Syndrome Foundation has advocated that the syndrome be renamed Willis-Ekbom disease.

Impact of RLS on Quality of Life and Morbidity

Fatigue is to be expected for people who have difficulty initiating and maintaining sleep. This, however, just touches the surface of the problem in individuals suffering with RLS. Many of these patients also have periodic motor limb disturbances whereby they make involuntary kicking and jerking movements, which may awaken them from sleep. In addition, these movements can disturb the sleep of the bed partner; it is not unusual for one to move to a different sleeping chamber, which may ultimately affect interpersonal relationships.

Morbidity of RLS is related to a higher incidence of hypertension, coronary artery disease, and stroke.[3] Whether this is due to hypoxia-driven inflammation during the sleep cycle or increased peripheral neurologic feedback and increased sympathetic tone is unknown.[4]

Current Pathophysiology of RLS

The precise etiology and pathophysiology of RLS are unknown. Current evidence revolves around dopaminergic dysfunction and altered control of iron homeostasis with CNS iron depletion.[5] Data for RLS-associated genetic links that allow for iron deficiency and other pathophysiological changes is also emerging.[6] Several risk polymorphisms (BTBD-9 [BTB (POZ) domain containing 9], MEIS-1 [Meis homeobox 1], protein tyrosine phosphatase, receptor type, D, and others) appear to play an important role and may interact or disturb dopaminergic and iron interactions.[7]

Peripheral neuropathy with or without clinical symptoms has long been proposed as a secondary cause for RLS in a number of disorders.[8]

Recently the endogenous opiate system has been suspected as having a role by stabilizing dopaminergic substantia nigra degeneration under conditions of iron deprivation. Interactions of endorphins and iron on the dopamine cell appear to be critical for adequate dopamine functioning. In a study by Sun and colleagues, application of enkephelin significantly protected the substantia nigra cells of mice from damage by iron deficiency.[9] The implications of this mouse model are that in RLS patients with iron deficiency, dopaminergic system dysfunction may result and an intact endogenous opioid system or opioid treatment may improve dopamine dysfunction. This theory is supported by a study examining autopsy tissue of RLS brains compared to controls. In this study there was a 37.5% reduction in beta-endorphin and met-enkephelin cells in the thalamus.[10] As a functional corollary to this research, a PET-scan study found regional negative correlations between endorphin binding and RLS severity in various parts of the brain—thus the lesser the degree of endorphin binding, the greater the severity of RLS symptoms.[11] This begets the theory that there may be a relative endorphin deficiency in RLS.

Alternative Theories for Pathophysiology of RLS

A recent controlled study demonstrated an increased prevalence of SIBO,[12] human immunodeficiency virus (HIV) infection, and systemic lupus erythematosus and RLS-associated cases with acute hepatitis C, *streptococcus* infection, *Mycoplasma* infection, and *Borrelia* infection, which suggest a potential role for inflammation and/or immunological disorders. Data to support that there is a direct attack on the CNS and peripheral nervous system (PNS) through humoral or cellular immune mechanisms are reported in a study by Matsuo in which antibodies against human caudate and putamen were identified in RLS patients with streptococcal and mycoplasma infections.[13]

In addition to SIBO, three other gastrointestinal disorders have recently been linked to RLS: liver disease, Crohn's disease, and celiac disease.[14] All three of these conditions can be associated with systemic inflammation, immune dysfunction, and SIBO, and may play a more general role in RLS.

The means by which inflammation and altered immunity could contribute to the cause and/or exacerbation of RLS includes three major theories: (1) inflammation causes CNS iron deficiency through alterations in hepcidin; (2) humoral or cellular immunological mechanisms cause a direct attack on the CNS or PNS; or (3) RLS gene variants interact with inflammatory disorders, immune alterations, and/or chronic infections such as SIBO to potentiate them.

The intestinal tract mucosa is frequently exposed to antigens, bacteria, and chemicals, and yet is selective about what is absorbed. An intact gut barrier is a complex system and depends on anatomic tight junctions, immune function, and antimicrobial chemicals. Bacterial overgrowth and enteric infections are two major insults to the gut that result in increased permeability and enteropathy via damage to the tight junctions of mucosal cells. When the gut is damaged, there is a subsequent increase in systemic inflammation.

In a review of forty-seven conditions associated with RLS, forty-two (89%) of these conditions were found to be associated with inflammation and/or immune changes.[15] The general division of these conditions can be grouped as neurological (seventeen), gastrointestinal (five), rheumatologic (seven), metabolic (six), pulmonary (five) and other varied conditions (seven). In the thirty-eight conditions where there were control groups to show that the condition was highly associated with RLS, thirty-six (95%) were associated with inflammation and/or immune changes. Inflammation was most commonly associated with elevated TNF-α levels and pro-inflammatory interleukins, predominantly interleukin-6, but also interleukins 1, 2, 4, 12, 17, and 18. Interleukin-17 has a unique role, and has been found to orchestrate the inflammatory response in inflammatory and auto-immune diseases of the nervous system, and in systemic diseases including rheumatoid arthritis. In addition, twenty-one (49%) of the conditions were associated with iron deficiency, eighteen (42%) with peripheral neuropathy, and fifteen (35%) with SIBO.

In primary and familial RLS, central iron deficiency is well documented by cerebrospinal fluid, magnetic resonance imaging, and autopsy studies.[16] Inflammation can lead to systemic iron deficiency, and it therefore seems reasonable that inflammation could trigger CNS iron deficiency and subsequent RLS symptoms. Hepcidin may be the primary link to explain this phenomenon. This peptide is the principal hormone involved in the regulation of iron levels, and has been shown to be produced by the liver in humans and by the brain in animal models.[17] It is known that increased hepcidin levels can lead to decreased serum iron levels, and perhaps decreased availability of iron to the brain. Increased hepcidin levels may occur in the setting of inflammation, as it is known that inflammation can lead to IL-6 production, which can stimulate hepcidin production. Additionally, in the setting of infection, lipopolysaccharides (LPSs) form as a breakdown product of bacteria, which are also known to stimulate hepcidin production.

Direct up-regulation of hepcidin production in the choroid plexus by systemic inflammation and LPS as seen in murine models could also explain CNS iron deficiency. In humans, a search for pro-hepcidin, a precursor to hepcidin, demonstrated increased levels in the brain tissue of early onset RLS patients, including neuromelanin cells, substantia nigra, and putamen, and decreased levels in the CSF. This suggests a potential role of hepcidin in primary RLS patients. Ferroportin has been demonstrated to be present on ependymal cells of the choroid plexus lining the ventricles. When hepcidin becomes bound to choroid plexus-associated ferroportin, this could decrease availability of iron for the CNS.

SIBO

In the majority of small intestinal diseases associated with SIBO (i.e., small bowel pseudo-obstruction, jejunal diverticulosis), systemic iron deficiency anemia due to malabsorption of iron from the duodenum is generally not a problem; thus, simple malabsorption is not a good explanation for how SIBO could lead to CNS iron deficiency. A more likely explanation is that cytokines or circulating lipopolysaccharides released in the setting of SIBO could induce hepcidin release with subsequent reduced transportation of iron into the choroid plexus and brain tissue as stated above. Circulating levels of cytokines such as TNF-α and pro-inflammatory interleukins are elevated in SIBO and in IBS. Recent evidence indicates that low-grade SIBO can present with virtually no gastrointestinal symptoms, but may affect the body in profound ways due to systemic inflammation and increased intestinal permeability. This is the critical concept that may tie together dysbiosis in the gut and unexplained syndromes and diseases.

In a recent study the lactulose breath test was used to diagnose SIBO in patients with primary RLS.[18] IBS and SIBO were reported to be highly associated with RLS. IBS was diagnosed in 28% of RLS subjects compared to 4% of controls (p > 0.0317). SIBO was diagnosed in 69% of RLS subjects compared to 28% of controls who were unselected for gastro-intestinal symptoms (p > 0.0033) and compared to 10% of completely asymptomatic controls.

Current Medical Therapy for RLS

In general, pharmacological treatment should be limited to those patients who have symptoms that impair the patient's quality of life, daytime functioning, social functioning, or sleep.[19] Intermittent "on demand" treatment is appropriate in some RLS patients, and includes carbidopa/levodopa, pramipexole, ropinirole, oxycodone, methadone, codeine, and tramadol. Patients who suffer from chronic RLS should be treated with either a dopamine agonist or an α-2-δ calcium channel ligand. The α-2-δ ligands include gabapentin, gabapentin enacarbil, and pregabalin. A dopamine agonist is preferred in the setting of depression and obesity. As α-2-δ ligands can alleviate chronic pain and may be helpful in treating anxiety and insomnia, the presence of any of these comorbidities may favor their use. For RLS present through much of the day and night, the use of long-acting agents, such as the rotigotine patch or gabapentin enacarbil, should be considered. In refractory RLS, oral prolonged-release oxyco-done-naloxone has been recommended.

A review of therapy by Hornyak and colleagues showed that virtually all treatments were comparable in reducing the severity score of RLS.[20] The most common measurement of severity is the international restless legs syndrome (IRLS) score: IRLS score is 0–40 based on the 4-point response to ten questions. In Hornyak and colleagues' review the improvement (lessening of symptoms) was -5.47 points for dopamine agonists, -5.12 points for anticonvulsants ($\alpha_2\delta$ ligands and levetiracetam), and -4.59 points for iron treatments. Although central iron deficiency clearly plays a role in the pathogenesis and severity of RLS, simply infusing it or taking it by mouth alone is generally inadequate as a treatment.[21] In this review of five studies, the one exception was the dialysis patients with RLS. On the other hand, iron deficiency should trigger an aggressive work-up to determine the etiology, which can include gastrointestinal blood loss or malabsorption.[22]

Pertinent to the discussion of LDN that will follow, European investigators examined the use of prolonged-release oxycodone-naloxone for treatment of severe RLS after other therapies had failed.[23] The study drug was oxycodone 5.0 mg, naloxone 2.5 mg, twice per day, which was up-titrated according to the investigator's opinion to a maximum of oxycodone 40 mg, naloxone 20 mg, twice per day; in the extension part of the study, all patients started on oxycodone 5.0 mg, naloxone 2.5 mg, twice per day, which was up-titrated to a maximum of oxycodone 40 mg, naloxone 20 mg, twice per day. In this randomized study, 132 patients took prolonged-release oxycodone-naloxone versus 144 who took placebo. The mean IRLS score at randomization was 31.6 (standard deviation [SD] 4.5); mean change after twelve weeks was -16.5 (SD 11.3) in the prolonged-release oxycodone-naloxone group and -9.4 (SD 10.9) in the placebo group (p < 0.0001). After the extension phase, mean sum score was 9.7 (SD 7.8). Possibly owing to the high dose ratio of naloxone to narcotic there were frequent treatment-related adverse events: 73% patients in the prolonged-release oxycodone-naloxone group versus 43% in the placebo group during the double-blind phase.

Discussion of Postinfectious Syndromes

The importance of postenteric infections causing systemic diseases and syndromes is paramount since there are approximately seventy-six million episodes of food poisoning per year in the United States.[24] Data from the Centers for Disease Control and Prevention (CDC) show that foodborne illnesses cause 325,000 hospitalizations and 5,000 deaths per year. Chronic disorders after these infections include hemolytic uremic syndrome, chronic renal disease, diabetes, reactive arthritis, Reiter's syndrome, and postinfectious IBS, which range from 7% to 34% after a bacterial infection.[25]

Immunologic mechanisms focus on either humoral or cellular immunity and include studies of antibodies, cellular immune disturbances, macrophages, natural killer cells, nitric oxide, and complement. Molecular mimicry is the most widely held belief explaining how bacteria or viruses can trigger autoimmune disorders, and this has roles in various diseases. The best example in neurological diseases, and one of the most severe postenteric complications, is Guillain Barré syndrome, which can occur after *Campylobacter* enteritis, especially in individuals with a specific genotype.[26]

One theory for RLS is that antigenic stimuli by gastrointestinal bacteria or antigens could result in autoimmune nerve damage in the CNS, spinal cord, or PNS, and result in RLS. Several diseases and syndromes associated with RLS highlight this possible hypothesis.

Case Study of Postinfectious Syndromes with RLS

The following case history illustrates what can be seen as a consequence of a foodborne illness and how gastrointestinal dysfunction may explain seemingly unrelated idiopathic syndromes.

The patient is a fifty-five-year-old Caucasian woman who was an intensive care unit nurse before she became disabled from her idiopathic syndromes. She had seen twelve physicians and alternative medical caregivers to diagnose and treat her conditions, which developed after a self-limited, acute, nonbloody diarrheal illness acquired at a restaurant twenty years prior. Soon after the infection she developed IBS with abdominal pain, bloating, and altered bowel movements. A year later she developed fibromyalgia with chronic fatigue and ultimately myalgias so severe that she was unable to touch her legs. She became disabled and had to quit her job. Her fatigue worsened eight years later when she noticed characteristic symptoms of RLS (the compelling urge to move the legs at night associated with leg discomfort). Her sleep was greatly impaired and her fatigue worsened. She fell asleep while driving and had a motor vehicle accident. Three years later she developed symptoms of urinary frequency and urgency, pelvic pain, and pain during intercourse.

The patient finally was tested for SIBO with a lactulose breath test. She noted rapid and sustained clinical improvement in all of her symptoms after two weeks of rifaximin, a nonabsorbable broad-spectrum antibiotic, followed by 4.5 mg naltrexone daily for the past six years.

Additional Cases of Restless Leg Syndrome with SIBO and LDN Therapy

A sixty-nine-year-old white female was seen for complaints of discomfort and restlessness in her legs. She reported an aching sensation with pulsation that occurred when lying down and would get better when moving and stretching her legs. Additional medical complaints included constipation, bloating, flatulence, bad breath, and fatigue. She had a two-week course of rifaximin for bacterial overgrowth as determined by a lactulose breath test. Two weeks after the first course of therapy she slept for two nights without RLS for the first time in many years. A second course of antibiotic therapy was administered and was followed by LDN. The use of 2.5 mg of naltrexone each morning has kept the RLS completely at bay for the past seven years. Her constipation continues to be a problem.

A sixty-three-year-old white female complained that for the previous three years she had suffered pain in her legs (experienced as muscle aches) whenever she lay down in bed, which interrupted her sleep. The pain was never present while walking. Similar pain was present when she was sitting still on an airplane. Touching or massaging her legs gave her discomfort. Other symptoms included constipation and halitosis. A lactulose breath test was administered, which revealed excess methane excretion. A course of rifaximin was given. She noted rapid relief of the leg symptoms. At that time she was on a statin medicine for high cholesterol, so LDN 2.5 mg at bedtime was prescribed, with the initial idea that it might increase her gastrointestinal motility and reduce recurrence of the SIBO. Over the ensuing years she has had two relapses of RLS symptoms. Repeating a course of rifaximin led to rapid relief, and the LDN was continued to minimize the potential for relapse.

Additional RLS cases where LDN was used as part of the protocol are summarized below.

Open Label Multimodality for RLS with SIBO

The first clinical trial of an antibiotic in the setting of RLS was in 2008. In this study 13 IBS patients who had SIBO and RLS demonstrated that 77% of the patients (10 of 13) had ≥80% long-lasting improvement of RLS symptoms following open-label treatment with rifaximin 1,200 mg/day for ten days. This treatment was followed by motility and probiotic therapy.[27] The motility therapy used in this study included low-dose erythromycin, which mimics the gastrointestinal hormone motilin and was designed to reduce the return of the SIBO. The probiotic used was a *Bifidobacterium* species, which may reduce inflammation and immune dysfunction on the gastrointestinal mucosa.

Results from Rifaximin Monotherapy Studies

The next study included patients with primary RLS who had a positive lactulose breath test for SIBO.[28] The mean baseline IRLS score was 23.1; the rating of RLS symptoms is based upon ten questions with a 0–4 scale on each. Open-label treatment with rifaximin 1,200 mg/day for ten days followed by 400 mg/every other day for twenty days resulted in a decrease in the IRLS score by 10.7 in 9 of 14 patients. Two of the five RLS nonresponders had improvement with a second course of rifaximin when combined with metronidazole, and a third patient improved when she was later diagnosed with celiac disease and placed on a gluten-free diet and iron supplementation.

The next monotherapy study was a double-blind study.[29] Patients were screened for SIBO using lactulose breath test. Patients with an abnormal lactulose breath test received rifaximin 550 mg thrice daily (n = 20) or placebo (n = 10) for ten days. The IRLS, global RLS symptoms, and gastrointestinal symptoms were assessed over twenty-five days. In the IRLS responders (i.e., patients with a positive change in IRLS scores), mean improvement in IRLS scores on day eleven was significantly greater for rifaximin (-6.0 ± 5.0) compared with placebo (1.7 ± 5.1; p = 0.017). Results from a similar analysis on day eighteen approached a statistically significant difference between groups (-7.8 ± 5.1 vs. -0.33 ± 10; p = 0.058). Rifaximin improved IRLS scores for all 20 patients from baseline to days eleven (p = 0.037) and eighteen (p = 0.006) compared with placebo. Maximal IRLS improvement for all rifaximin patients showed a numeric positive trend compared with that of the placebo group (-4.5 ± 6.6 vs. -0.6 ± 8.0; p = 0.130). Marked and moderate global improvement of RLS symptoms occurred in 40% and 22% of patients in the rifaximin and placebo groups, respectively. Gastrointestinal symptoms improved more with rifaximin than with placebo.

These two monotherapy studies contrast with what was seen in the author's general practice by following antibiotic therapy with additional modalities to reduce inflammation and improve gastrointestinal motility. In light of the concerns that inflammation was a contributing factor to RLS in the CNS, the investigators began to offer LDN to their patients. The result of this therapeutic endeavor appeared to be good and is discussed below.

Results from Retrospective LDN Study in SIBO-Positive and SIBO-Negative Patients

Patients who were prescribed LDN for RLS from 2006 to 2014 had their chart reviewed. In total, 52 patient charts were reviewed. Ten patients were eliminated from further analysis for the following reasons: They did not fill their prescription, they did not have a follow-up appointment and were lost to follow-up, or they did not fulfill all criteria for RLS. In the remaining 42 patients, 23 received 2.5 mg once daily, 10 received 2.5 mg twice daily, and 9 received 4.5 mg daily.

The clinical characteristics of the 42 patients who were followed included: mean age fifty-eight years, ratio of 38:4, and mean body mass index of 27.1 kilograms per square millimeter (kg/mm²). Duration of LDN administration was a mean of 76.5 weeks (range 1–348). All but three patients had a lactulose breath test; in the 39 who had the test, 30 (77%) had a positive test for SIBO. A total of 35 of the 42 (83%) were treated with antibiotic therapy before the administration of LDN. The outcome was determined by review of the chart or, when unsure, contacting the patient. The assessment grossly determined if their RLS symptoms were markedly better, moderately better, slightly better, unchanged, or worsened. They were also asked if they had side effects and if these led to cessation of the medication.

The results of this retrospective study were that LDN with and without antibiotic therapy led to a RLS state that was markedly better in 21, moderately better in 5, slightly better in 2, and unchanged in 13 patients. Comparing the low dose to higher dose of LDN, it appeared that a higher proportion did better on 2.5 mg daily than the higher doses: The 2.5 mg dose group was markedly better in 15, moderately better in 3, slightly better in 0, and unchanged in 5 versus the higher dose groups who were markedly better in 6, moderately better in 2, slightly better in 3, and unchanged in 8. Examining the 7 patients who received LDN without antibiotic therapy, the following was observed: RLS was markedly better in 1, moderately better in 2, slightly better in 1, and unchanged in 3. Finally, 22 patients with marked to moderate response were helped in the maintenance phase for a mean of 107 weeks (range 4–348 weeks, SD 118). The outcome data is shown in table 6.1.

TABLE 6.1. Outcome of Patients Treated with LDN with and without Antibiotics for RLS

	Markedly better	Moderately better	Slightly better	Unchanged
All patients (N = 42)	21	5	3	13
2.5 mg LDN (N = 23)	15	3	0	5
4.5 – 5.0 mg LDN (N = 19)	6	2	3	8
LDN without antibiotic (N = 7)	1	2	1	3

Adverse events led to cessation of LDN in 6 of 42 (14%) of the patients. The 6 were equally divided in those who received the lower (2.5 mg) and higher (4.5–5 mg) doses. Of those 6 patients, 5 were getting clinical benefit but had to stop nonetheless.

Summary

More work remains to be done before we can recommend LDN to RLS patients. Various questions need to be addressed. With regard to the role in therapy, is LDN the drug best used for maintenance of SIBO treatment or can it be used for primary therapy? Concerns for pathophysiology are addressed by questions that include: Does it exert effect through improving SIBO via motility, does it change central or peripheral nerve pain via toll-like receptors and reduce neuroinflammation, and does it improve endorphin activity and hence improve dopamine nerve function in the setting of iron deficiency?

A double-blind, placebo-controlled study must be performed. Although this would ideally include patients with SIBO who have been treated with antibiotics first, it will be hard to determine the impact of the LDN since many patients seem to have immediate improvement with antibiotic treatment alone. It seems unlikely that antibiotic therapy could be implied to have a very long action alone. Alternatively, a double-blind study of LDN alone may show blunted results if the triggering factor is not treated first. Nonetheless, individuals appear to have had remarkable responses to LDN for long-term prevention of a disorder that rarely goes into spontaneous remission.

SEVEN

Depression

Mark Shukhman, MD
and Rebecca Shukhman

Any substance that can increase the amount of endorphins in the body can find an application in psychiatry. The vast majority of the low dose naltrexone (LDN) literature, however, is written about the benefits in treatments of somatic illnesses. Perhaps this is because both patients and doctors get caught up in focusing on the "big illness," on monitoring test results and MRI scans, forgetting that quality of life starts with how people feel and think and how they can adjust to changes in their lives caused by illness.

Experience shows that while psychiatrists are more likely to label the symptoms of comorbid psychiatric conditions correctly, most primary care practitioners and, notably, specialists, tend to see emotional suffering as "appropriate in the circumstances." In the language of psychodynamic psychiatry, these doctors are not trained to be constantly aware of their countertransference. This simply means that doctors frequently make assumptions (about a patient's emotional state, for example) by imagining themselves in their patient's place and assuming that the patient has the same feelings as they would have, should they end up with the same illness and circumstances.

Depression in the General Population and Among Patients with Chronic Illnesses

Depression is a common illness, even in the general population, with women affected approximately twice as often as men. In the United States, depression affects at least 12% of women and 8% of men in their lifetimes.

In some countries, the reported rate is even higher. Among patients with serious medical conditions, the rate of depression is significantly higher, approaching at least one third. Depression frequently co-occurs with chronic illnesses and can actually be considered one of the most common complications of chronic illness. Nevertheless, it is not frequently recognized and even less frequently addressed as a separate condition by either patients or their doctors. This may be partly because many of the symptoms of depression, such as fatigue, insomnia, and poor appetite, may also represent the symptoms of a chronic medical illness, and partly because medical doctors are not attuned to recognizing psychiatric conditions. Some doctors may feel that the patient won't take them seriously or that the patient will feel that the doctor is minimizing their "real symptoms" if they talk about moods, anxiety, feelings, and behaviors, rather than about test results and MRI pictures. Such symptoms as intense sadness, loss of interest in previously enjoyable activities, rumination about the changes in life, loss of future potential, and pessimism, are more likely to be seen by the doctors treating a medical condition as "a normal reaction to having a serious illness," rather than a hint to start an evaluation for possible associated depression. The attitude that "anybody would feel the same in such a situation" prevails among medical doctors treating patients with chronic illnesses.

An alternative approach is to recognize the combination of a medical illness and depression as a "double burden." Research has shown that people with chronic medical illnesses that are complicated by depression experience not only worsened quality of life and more complications during the course of the illness but also worse outcomes. This is unfortunate because at least one of the conditions of that double burden—depression—is frequently very treatable. Treating depression is crucial for the best outcome. It helps the patient to better cope with the general medical illness, to seek treatment and tolerate that treatment, to not be discouraged by setbacks, and to adjust to the living of a quality life, albeit with limitations imposed by the illness.

Modern psychiatry does not offer a reliable "test" for depression. The patient is determined to have a major depressive disorder if he or she has a certain number of symptoms from the list provided in the most recent *Diagnostic and Statistical Manual of Mental Disorders (DSM-5)*. On one hand, labeling a condition based on a certain well-described criteria helps, for example, to guide the selection of patients for research. If a medication

SYMPTOMS OF MAJOR DEPRESSIVE DISORDER[1]

For at least two weeks:

- Depressed mood and/or lack of interest or pleasure

Plus at least four of the following:

- Significant weight loss or gain
- Sleeping too much or too little
- Slowed thinking or movement that is noticeable to others
- Fatigue or low energy nearly every day
- Feeling of worthlessness or inappropriate guilt
- Loss of concentration or indecisiveness
- Recurrent thoughts of death or suicide

is shown to be effective, for example for "major depressive disorder," it tells the clinician that a patient with the cluster of symptoms listed in that book and combined under a specific name—"major depressive disorder" in this case—is likely to improve on that medication. On the other hand, a method of establishing a diagnosis based on the constellation of symptoms likely leads to aggregation of multiple different illnesses with heterogeneous mechanisms and even manifestations, course, prognosis, and treatment options into the same category.

Depression or Chronic Illness?

Recognizing the presence of a mood disorder in circumstances where someone is struggling to adjust to loss of health and, hence, the need to make adjustments to plans for the future is frequently a difficult task.

It is natural for such a patient to have waves of sadness and feelings of emptiness and loss, especially following thoughts or reminders of this loss. In the presence of a depressive illness, however, sadness becomes persistent, with an inability to anticipate happiness or pleasure; it is not tied to specific thoughts or preoccupations. The person is constantly in a state of unhappiness and misery. In a "normal reaction to illness," pain and grief may be accompanied by positive emotions and humor; self-esteem is preserved and

TABLE 7.1. Differentiating Major Depressive Disorder from a Normal Reaction to Illness

Reaction to Illness	Major Depressive Disorder
Feeling of emptiness and loss	Persistent depressed mood, inability to anticipate happiness or pleasure
Dysphoria occurs in waves, triggered by thoughts or reminders of the loss; decreases over time	Depressed mood is more persistent; not tied to specific thoughts or preoccupations
Pain or grief may be accompanied by positive emotions and humor	Pervasive unhappiness and misery
Preoccupation with thoughts about changes in life related to disease	Pessimistic, self-critical ruminations
Preserved self-esteem	Feeling of worthlessness and self-loathing
Derogatory ideations typically involve perceived failings related to solving the problem	Suicidal ideations related to feeling worthless, undeserving of life, or unable to cope with the pain of depression

negative self-perception is related to the perceived failings related to solving the problems. In depression, the patient is constantly pessimistic and has self-critical ruminations with feelings of worthlessness and self-loathing. Normal reactions to illness are not accompanied by suicidal ideations, related to a feeling of worthlessness and of being undeserving of life or an inability to cope with the pain of depression (table 7.1).

LDN as a Psychiatric Medication

Some of the psychiatric benefits of LDN, such as improvements in fatigue and in psychomotor activity, are commonly mentioned as target symptoms for the treatment of other somatic conditions, especially with overlapping symptomatology, such as in fibromyalgia, multiple sclerosis, and lupus, among others. Great results have been seen in the treatment of such psychiatric conditions as autism spectrum disorder, posttraumatic stress disorder (PTSD), and personality disorders, especially dissociative disorders (depersonalization/derealization, as seen in PTSD; dissociative amnesia; and dissociative identity disorder, better known as multiple personalities disorder).

There is, however, also practical experience and research looking into the use of LDN in depression, anxiety, obsessive-compulsive disorder, psychosis, and even in the modification of sex drive. Some other reported uses include the management of insomnia, narcolepsy, restless legs syndrome, dementia, schizophrenia, self-injuring behavior, impulse-control behaviors, and bulimia. LDN can be used in addiction for the purpose of extinguishing unwanted behaviors. While naltrexone is approved by the FDA for the treatment of alcohol and opioid dependence in traditional doses, in our practice we were able to modify the officially recommended strategy to the use of naltrexone in *low* doses for alcoholism, addiction to stimulants, addiction to food, and the treatment of so-called "process addictions," for example Internet use, gambling, sex, and food. In our practice, we also created a treatment for alcohol addiction that modifies the well-proven Sinclair Method of strategically timed standard doses of naltrexone to the use of LDN.

What Makes LDN a Psychiatric Medication?

LDN increases the release of opioid peptides, which is a collective name for endorphins, enkephalins, dynorphins, and other psychoactive substances, produced by our body. This clearly makes it relevant to psychiatry. LDN can help decrease fatigue and other somatic symptoms. Often this alone can help the patient feel better and perhaps be less depressed. LDN is frequently reported to cause vivid dreams, which implies that it can change sleep architecture. Modifying sleep architecture by itself can modify many psychiatric conditions.[2] For example, REM sleep deprivation is a well-known strategy for the treatment of major depressive disorder. Despite ongoing research and practical evidence, it has not yet become common knowledge that depression is also linked to various immunological conditions.[3] The anti-inflammatory properties of LDN can assist in recovery from depression. In our practice, LDN is also used for medication-enhanced psychotherapy. It helps to extinguish unwanted feelings, thoughts, and behaviors, while we as doctors are focusing on those feelings, thoughts, and behaviors we want to enhance.

LDN and Opioid Receptors

Most of the time, when the LDN literature discusses the role of LDN in increasing endorphins, it goes on to talk about the role of endorphins in autoimmune conditions, inflammation, tissue repair, and so on, and circumvents the role of endorphins *as endorphins*, which are psychoactive substances to begin with. We produce endorphins naturally in response to exercise, orgasm, pain, food (such as chocolate, spices, alcohol), fear (this is why kids like scary movies), compulsive behaviors, touch, smell, sunshine, and other pleasurable activities. The word *endorphin* itself is a combination of the words *endogenous* and *morphine*, owing to the fact that it is produced in our bodies and acts as an opiate. The majority of the applications of LDN focus on its effects on the immune system, forgetting that endorphins also make us feel fuzzy and warm when we fall in love; help us in times of physical and emotional stress; and bring us joy, contentment, and feelings of general well-being.

Although there is no reliable way to measure the level of endorphins in our bodies and there is no official definition for "endorphin deficiency," we can compare the experiences of people coming off methadone (this is an example of when an externally given opioid is removed) or people who say they "suddenly understood what it meant to feel normal" when they were first introduced to opiates, to describe the sensation. In addition to the obvious symptoms of withdrawal, people coming off methadone describe depression, insomnia, increased body aches and pains, and loss of sense of humor and feelings of pleasure. They have no interest in previously enjoyable activities long after the withdrawal is over. Due to the lack of a clear definition and distinct research on the matter, one can find multiple opinions about what endorphin deficiency looks like. A person with endorphin deficiency has been described as uncomfortable due to the slightest disturbances in the surroundings—changes in sound, light, temperature, or touch (so-called "sensory defensiveness"). Endorphin deficiency is often accompanied by immunological problems such as frequent colds, allergies, and autoimmune conditions. People with endorphin deficiency might not have the experience of a so-called "runner's high," they may cry easily or be extremely sensitive to emotional or physical pain, and they may generally avoid dealing with painful life issues. They crave pleasures, comfort, reward, chocolate, wine, marijuana, and tobacco.[4] By providing additional endorphins or by increasing sensitivity of receptors to endorphins, LDN can be effective for relieving these symptoms of endorphin deficiency.

Opioid Receptors in the Expression of Psychiatric Symptoms

The use of LDN results in increased levels of endogenous opioids: endorphins, enkephalins, and deltorphins. These, in turn, activate the three main opioid receptors in the body, named mu, kappa, and delta, each with a unique significance in psychiatry.

The mu receptors, activated by beta-endorphins and enkephalins, are linked not only to pain modulation but also to euphoria and sedation experienced by the users of opiates. Activation of these receptors also leads to an increase in GABA, the effect sought by the users of Valium, Xanax, or alcohol.

The kappa receptor is especially sensitive to the subset of endogenous opioids called dynorphins. The role of these receptors is implicated in stress-related depression and anxiety. These receptors also play an important role in addiction. Overactivation of kappa receptors, as seen, for example, in opioid withdrawal, causes dysphoria, body aches, anxiety, and depression. Kappa receptors can be activated with salvinorin A, ibogane, ketamine, and pentazocine. In our practice, we have used these substances to ease opioid withdrawal because of their role in addiction-control mechanisms. Naltrexone is an FDA-approved treatment of opioid dependence. Because it is an opioid (mu and kappa) receptor blocker, it can be given only after a patient's body is free of opioids, which means that they have to go through opioid withdrawal. By the time naltrexone can be started, the craving for an opioid becomes very intense. This is perhaps the reason why most patients refuse naltrexone (ReVia, Vivitrol) treatment. They assume that by taking an opioid blocker they will no longer be able to relapse, even if the craving becomes intolerable. They are partially right: Naltrexone blocks the mu receptors, which prevent opioids such as heroin from "working." They do not realize, however, that, by also blocking the kappa receptors, with naltrexone the cravings can be expected to significantly attenuate or disappear.

Blocking kappa receptors may be beneficial for the treatment of depression. There is no medication that can do it without also activating the mu receptor, which is associated with all the negative qualities of narcotics: "getting high," tolerance, dependence, and addiction. The solution again comes from naltrexone. The combination of buprenorphine (found in Bunavail, Buprenex, Suboxone, Subutex, and Zubsolv), a very potent kappa antagonist and partial mu agonist, with naltrexone, which blocks the unwanted effects of buprenorphine on mu receptors, is being studied as a novel antidepressant combination therapy.

The delta receptors are activated by enkephalins and deltorphins. Activation of these receptors can decrease symptoms of depression. A new drug in development,[5] at this point still without a name and referred to as RB-101, inhibits the breakdown and thus increases the available amount of enkephalins, providing not only analgesic, but also anxiolytic and antidepressant effects.[6] Activation of delta receptors can also increase the production of brain-derived neurotrophic factor (BDNF),[7] which has become one of the most frequent targets for recent psychiatric research.[8] Conditions linked to decreased BDNF include depression, bipolar disorder, obsessive-compulsive disorder, schizophrenia, anorexia nervosa, and bulimia, as well as autism spectrum disorders and dementias, including Alzheimer's disease. There is also a link between BDNF and addiction. BDNF-level modification with LDN can possibly decrease the risk of addiction. During the last few years, multiple studies have been published showing that depression leads to brain (specifically, hippocampal) atrophy.[9] BDNF was named as one of the factors that is protective against this atrophy. This fact essentially provides the evidence that depression can change both the function of the brain and the structure of the brain. It tells us that not only some of the autoimmune or neurological conditions that many LDN users are suffering from but also long-standing depression can lead to structural changes related to the loss of brain cells. This finding further emphasizes the need to recognize depression and treat it as an issue separate from the "main illness." If addressing depression can decrease brain atrophy, it is a good reason to take it seriously and treat it aggressively.

Another example of changes in the brain related to emotional experiences can be found in research linking decreased level of BDNF to childhood abuse, trauma, and other adverse psychological early life experiences.[10] It is well known that childhood trauma leads to psychiatric problems later in life. Before this research was conducted, the link between trauma and later psychiatric problems was attributed to emotional dysregulation and to various ineffective learned strategies that remain rigid despite proving to be maladaptive. This research essentially changed our view by pointing out that adverse, traumatic emotional experiences in early life lead not only to emotional and behavioral disturbances but also to structural changes in the brain that might persist for the rest of a person's life. BDNF can not only decrease the amount of brain atrophy, but might also repair some of the structural changes in the brain.

Besides LDN, BDNF can also be increased by glutamine, curcumin, exercise, cannabidiol (an orphan drug, Epidiolex, based on cannabidiol, is

FDA-approved for a rare form of childhood epilepsy), and tetrahydrocan-nabinol (THC—Marinol, based on THC, is an FDA-approved medication for AIDS-related anorexia). Intermittent fasting and calorie restriction—the same strategies that can prolong lifespan and decrease the likelihood of dementia—can also increase BDNF. Stress, on the other hand, can lower the amount of BDNF (as well as damage our brains and shorten our lives).

Anti-inflammatory Effects of LDN

In addition to its effect on opioid receptors, naltrexone has also been shown to interact with nonopioid receptors, such as toll-like receptor 4 (TLR4). These receptors are found on macrophages such as microglia, the immune cells in the central nervous system.[11] In other chapters of this book, you will find various implications of the anti-inflammatory effect of LDN on the somatic and mostly autoimmune illnesses. Besides immunomodulation, these receptors facilitate a cluster of psychiatric symptoms described collectively as "sickness behavior." These symptoms include not only somatic effects such as pain sensitivity, fatigue, and general malaise, but also cognitive disruption, sleep disorders, and mood disorders.[12] By antagonizing the TLR4 receptors, LDN can modify these psychosomatic phenomena. LDN has become a primary example of a relatively new class of therapeutic agents called glial cell modulators.[13]

LDN in the Treatment of Depression

Because naltrexone in "traditional doses" blocks opioid receptors, multiple psychiatric symptoms are mentioned as side effects in the package insert. Before turning to the evidence for the usefulness of LDN in the treatment of depression, we'll consider whether naltrexone in low doses can be expected to cause depression.

Does LDN Cause Depression?

From both theoretical and practical standpoints, it should not. The opioid receptor is exposed to LCN for a very short amount of time, not long enough for the effect of the blocked endorphin receptors to cause depression. Moreover, the short duration of opioid-receptor blockade is followed by an increase in endorphins, which is expected to improve mood and general well-being. As we will show later, the anti-immune and anti-inflammatory properties would also be more likely to alleviate depression than to cause it. In summary, from a theoretical standpoint, LDN is not expected to cause depression.

An increase in depression is also not seen in practice. Most of the research, looking even at the use of the traditional "high" doses of naltrexone for the treatment of opioid or alcohol addiction, schizophrenia, autism spectrum disorder, and other conditions, also does not show an increase in the incidence of depression.[14] The conclusions of most of these studies are similar to one published in 2006: "The results of the study suggest that depression *need not* be considered as a common adverse effect of naltrexone treatment or a treatment contraindication and that engaging with or adhering to naltrexone treatment may be associated with fewer depressive symptoms."[15]

What Makes LDN Useful in the Treatment of Depression?

There is no single theory explaining the mechanism of depression. It is very likely that various mechanisms produce the symptoms that can be clustered into the syndrome called depression. It is also important to remember that patients who meet the criteria for depression may have very different clinical presentations and different combinations of symptoms. A patient who reports feeling that his thought process is slowed, complains of sleeping too much and eating too much, is staying at home because he does not want to see anyone, and feels that his "thoughts are empty," meets the criteria for the diagnosis of major depressive disorder. A patient with a very different presentation, who reports having a lot of "nervous energy," is constantly worrying, is unable to fall asleep and wakes up earlier than expected, is losing appetite and weight, and who cannot concentrate because so many things are going through his mind, likely has a different mechanism of his illness, but also fits into the current criteria for major depressive disorder.[16] LDN can modify at least several of the mechanisms causing depression: neurotransmitters, opioid receptors, and inflammation.

Antidepressant Effects of LDN Related to Opioid-Receptor Activity

From what we know about endorphins, it seems logical to assume that they play a role in the alleviation of depression. The research supports this intuitive assumption. In the 1980s and 1990s, there were a number of studies showing significant improvement in depression and, in some cases, even the induction of temporary mania when depressed patients received injections of endorphins.[17] There is an interesting research theory that points to the importance of the opioid system in the mechanism of action of tricyclic antidepressants, medications usually associated with serotonergic activity. The theory is based on the observation that naltrexone, an opioid blocker, can reverse the antidepressant effects of the old tricyclic antidepressant imipramine.[18] Even though the efficacy of tricyclic antidepressants is traditionally associated with their serotonergic activity, the fact that imipramine is blocked by an opioid-receptor antagonist, naltrexone, means that opioid-like activity is involved in the mechanism of action of these medications.

To study depression, researchers use a number of standard animal models thought to correspond to depression in humans. For example, if a medication causes a caged animal to start pacing along the perimeter of the cage and to avoid the open space in the middle, this change in behavior is assumed to correspond to an increase in anxiety in a human. Another model compares "learned helplessness" in animals with depression in humans. To quantify depression, the researchers use the "forced swimming test." In this test, a rat is forced to swim until it "gives up." The hypothesis states that the less depressed the rat is, the longer it will swim. It was shown in multiple studies that a rat pretreated with an antidepressant does not give up as easily as an untreated rat. The opioid theory of depression is supported by the observation that blocking these rats' opioid receptors with naltrexone would negate the improvement in swimming time achieved by antidepressants.

Other research has implicated static or even increased levels of endorphins in the pathogenesis of depression, not decreased levels. This seeming contradiction can be resolved however, when we recognize the link between depression and the number of receptors, or—even better—the sensitivity of the receptors, not simply the level of endorphins circulating in the body. A similar theory is already accepted regarding serotonergic receptors, which are the targets for the serotonin-modulating antidepressants. Antidepressant medications can increase serotonin levels almost immediately, while alleviation of depressive symptoms takes time. The contemporary theory explains this by linking the decrease in depression not to the level of serotonin itself, but to the resultant changes in the receptors exposed to the elevated level of serotonin or, possibly, to the same genetic processes that lead to the down-regulation of receptors exposed to altered levels of serotonin.

No matter what the theory says, my patients on LDN like talking about "resetting the receptors to their previous healthy functioning."

Enhancing endorphins can assist in treatment of depression. Massage, acupuncture, sex, exercise, and other activities can increase endorphins temporarily. To achieve a more sustained increase, LDN, along with vitamins, supplements, and dietary changes, can be used. Dietary changes include a high-protein diet, preferably without sugar, flour, and coffee (the "exorphins"). In addition, vitamin B, vitamin C, omega-3 with vitamin D, vitamin E, zinc, capsaicin, and D-phenylalanine (up to 2,000 mg, three times a day) can be used. Recommendations also include minimizing stress and chronic pain and avoiding a sedentary lifestyle.

The Anti-inflammatory Pathway of the Antidepressant Effects of LDN

The link between depression and inflammation has been on the radar of researchers and drug companies for some time. Years ago, doctors studying neurosyphilis noted that later consequences of this infective illness were often associated with psychiatric symptoms, and they suspected that the immune system might be involved in the pathophysiology of depression. Other evidence supporting the inflammatory involvement in depression originates from the observation that immune-therapy treatment, such as interferon for hepatitis, is strongly associated with affective and behavioral changes, such as fatigue, lethargy, psychomotor slowness, poor concentration, reduction in grooming, loss of appetite and thirst, decreased interest in sex, depressed mood, hopelessness, anhedonia, social isolation, and suicidal ideations.[19] It has also been suggested that sickness behaviors could be induced by bacterial endotoxins. In one study,[20] it was shown that depressive symptoms were produced as soon as three hours after a typhoid injection. In the 1960s, an observation was made that the blood of sick animals can induce sickness behavior in other animals independently of the bacterial toxins.[21] In the 1980s, it was shown that this phenomenon is determined by cytokines, the products of activated leukocytes, and that depression induced by these inflammatory substances is not dissimilar from idiopathic major depression.[22] Moreover, it was shown that inhibition of cytokines and their signaling pathways has been associated with improved mood and with increased responsiveness to conventional antidepressant medications.[23]

To further point out that such depression is not a psychological reaction to being sick, we need to mention that sickness behavior is not unique to humans. Sick animals have very similar manifestations of illness, and pet owners can see when their pets become sick. They notice reduction in exploration (a dopamine-determined behavior), difference in social interaction (a serotonin-determined behavior), and difference in operant behaviors for food rewards, to name only a few examples. These behaviors are possibly adaptive in nature. Limiting movements could be explained by the need to conserve energy in order to raise temperature, anorexia might reduce the nutrition that feeds bacteria in the gut, lower threshold for pain limits the pressure on inflamed tissues, reduced grooming reduces water loss since licking the fur requires a lot of water, and so on.

Many antidepressant medications themselves have anti-inflammatory properties, not only peripherally, but also centrally, in microglia—the same place where LDN works.[24] This means that LDN works synergistically with antidepressant medications. It is possible that the doses of many medications (SSRIs, SNRIs, etc.) could be decreased with the addition of LDN to the treatment regimen.[25] For this reason, I frequently recommend LDN not only to my depressed patients with such inflammatory conditions as lupus, Crohn's disease, and ulcerative colitis, but also to patients with no known inflammatory conditions.

The Role of LDN as Dopamine Enhancer in Depression

So far, we have been following the consequences of the direct action of LDN on opioid receptors and on nonopioid receptors, such as TLR4 in the microglia. The role of LDN as a dopamine enhancer is a consequence of the further cascade of events triggered by the direct effects of LDN on opioid receptors. The beta-endorphins, produced in the arcuate nucleus of the brain, stimulate dopamine release in the nucleus accumbens directly and also indirectly by inhibiting GABA production in the ventral tegmental area. It is well known that opiates or endogenous opioids such as endorphins are associated with pleasurable feelings. This is achieved via dopamine release and GABA inhibition. In some people, this mechanism becomes "trained." For example, it has been shown that the release of beta-endorphins and dopamine is greater in patients with alcohol dependence relative to healthy controls.[26]

Dopamine release is known to produce pleasurable feelings—this is what stimulants such as cocaine do. But does dopamine play a role in alleviating depression? For a long time the pharmaceutical industry focused on the serotonergic theory of depression: serotonin, not dopamine, was the target for intervention. Thanks to this theory, we have such successful antidepressants as fluoxetine (Prozac), sertraline (Zoloft), citalopram/escitalopram (Celexa/Lexapro), fluvoxamine (Luvox), paroxetine (Paxil), and the most recent additions, vilazodone (Viibryd) and vortioxetine (Brintellix). The serotonergic theory, however, is only one of many, and not the first to have been offered. Originally, research focused on catecholamines (norepinephrine, epinephrine, and dopamine). Catecholamines are what wake you up, focus your brain, and put color into your day. Without enough catecholamines, life is gray, boring, and disorganized. When the limitations of the serotonergic drugs became obvious, the industry looked back and developed a number of medications, such as venlafaxine (Effexor), duloxetine (Cymbalta), desvenalfaxine (Pristiq), and the latest, levomilnacipran (Fetzima), which target not only serotonin, but also norepinephrine.

Dopamine in psychiatry has mostly been researched in relation to psychosis. This neurotransmitter, however, also plays a significant role in depression. Most of the disorders associated with dopamine deficiency are also associated with depression. Parkinson's disease is probably the most known example. Reserpine, an old medication once prescribed for the treatment of high blood pressure and psychosis, is a classic example of an effective medication that was forgotten because of the significant general, as well as psychiatric, side effects. The antihypertensive effect of reserpine was achieved by the rapid depletion of catecholamines. Unfortunately, the same depletion of catecholamines caused depression. Patients with schizophrenia, a dopamine-related illness, frequently show signs of so-called "negative symptoms," which have a lot in common with depression. Some studies have shown a correlation between the central nervous system's level of dopamine metabolites and psychomotor activity.[27] The mental and physical slowness that we see not only in Parkinson's disease or in Alzheimer's, but also in depression, is likely related to the low level of dopamine.[28]

Increasing catecholamines, on the other hand, can help alleviate depression. A very strong catecholamine-releasing drug, cocaine, improves mood, although only initially and only for a short time. After a while, the effect turns into its opposite, the "crash" (from catecholamine depletion) and results in even deeper depression. Multiple efforts have been devoted to creating a longer-acting stimulant that does not produce a "crash." Psychostimulants like dextroamphetamine, methylphenidate, and others would release catecholamines and are known to improve depression, in some cases alone or, most effectively, when added to antidepressant medications. The "wakefulness promoting agent," modafinil, (or its newest modification armodafinil) is far from cocaine and even from stimulants in terms of the intensity of stimulation, but, at the same time, is not causing withdrawals. Unlike stimulants, which work by "opening the gates" for the exchange of the ions between the cell and intracellular space, this medication "keeps the gates half-open," thus facilitating the constant action and preventing the neurotransmitters from rapid depletion.[29]

One of the newer, less likely to be abused stimulants, lisdexamfetamine (Vyvanse), has come close to receiving an official FDA approval for the treatment of patients who failed to improve from two or more antidepressants.

Catecholamines can also be increased with another, infrequently used class of old antidepressants called monoamine oxidase inhibitors (MAOI). Even greater increases in catecholamines can be achieved with the combined use of stimulants and MAOI.[30] Unfortunately, prescribing these combinations often results in multiple panicked phone calls from the pharmacy, because the combination would trigger the "major contraindication" warning on their computers. I am not advocating this combination to prescribers without experience, but I do believe it's one of the best antidepressant combinations, effective because of its robust increase in the release of catecholamines. Last, direct dopaminergic drugs such as L-dopa and others used in Parkinson's disease have had positive effects in the treatment of depression. They are not routinely used for depression, however, because of multiple side effects, which may include hypersexuality and problematic gambling.

Many commonly used antidepressants can increase dopamine. Wellbutrin represents a group called norepinephrine and dopamine reuptake inhibitors (NDRIs). Another medication from the same group, nomifensine, with cheerfully sounding brand names Merital and Alival, was available for a short time as a very effective antidepressant.[31] Many common antidepressants not normally associated with dopaminergic activity, such as nefazodone, mirtazapine, doxepin, venlafaxine, duloxetine, and even Zoloft in higher doses, also increase dopamine.

Adding LDN to the Depression Treatment Regime

To summarize the above, LDN—via both opioid and nonopioid receptors, and via direct and indirect actions—modulates inflammatory response and the level of endogenous opioids and dopamine. Though this may be just the tip of the iceberg, even these few mechanisms can give us guidance to the potential use of LDN in psychiatry. Treating depression with LDN produces great results, and the effect of the treatment is shown to be independent from the improvement in the general medical condition that the depression frequently accompanies. Although in some cases depression can be treated with LDN alone, most of the cases we see in our office are already considered "treatment resistant" by the standards of the field, and thus by the time of the initial presentation the patients are already taking multiple medications. Stopping their medications and introducing LDN alone would not be prudent and in some cases might even be dangerous. Consequently, most of our experience is in using LDN as an add-on treatment.

Who is an appropriate patient for LDN augmentation or monotherapy? The research does not give us guidance about "matching the medication to a right patient" or about the choice of one medication versus another. The official guidelines focus on avoiding potential specific side effects of medications rather than on targeting specific symptoms. Though much attention in this chapter has been dedicated to inflammation, and to opioid and dopamine related depressions, it is important to recognize that even if depression seems to be "serotonin related," LDN still can be effective. One explanation is that receptors pretreated with serotonin are more sensitive to dopamine.[32] We have had successful cases when depression that previously did not respond to an SSRI (a class of medications that are considered to be purely serotonergic) was improved simply with the addition of LDN.

As mentioned already, there are no clear guidelines to determine whether depression is related to decreased serotonin or decreased dopamine. The imbalance of neurotransmitters, rather than deficiency of one of them, matters the most. It is also important to remember that the majority of depressions are multifactorial, and imbalance of the neurotransmitters is just a part of the mechanism. Nevertheless, when choosing an appropriate target, consciously or subconsciously, we are trying to guess which system is deficient.

Dopamine-Deficient Depression

Dopamine is involved in pleasure and reward; in memory and motor control; in activation, arousal, and cognition; and in reward-motivating behavior. Dopamine facilitates attachment and love and altruism; it also helps to integrate thoughts and feelings. Consequently, depressed people with a predominantly low dopamine level complain of a loss of satisfaction; chronic boredom; apathy; no attachment and love; no remorse; and difficulties concentrating, focusing, remembering, and thinking abstractly. They oversleep, have no motivation, procrastinate, and report that pleasures feel dull and that their libido is decreased. They may zone out in front of the television, be less interested in social relationships, and have decreased eye contact; they are detail-oriented and not looking at the whole picture; they may become quick to anger and even cruel. They avoid exercising, but tend to crave caffeine, sugar, alcohol, and saturated fats—unfortunately, the same foods that can further lower their dopamine level. Dopamine-deficient patients are more likely to have restless legs syndrome and, in severe cases, may even look "parkinsonian," that is, physically and mentally slowed, with decreased facial expression and monotone voice. For patients with a predominantly dopamine-depletion-related depression, we use LDN along with medications that likely increase dopamine levels. These medications include amantadine, psychostimulants, buproprion, high doses of mirtazapine, and MAOIs. At the same time, excessive flooding of the receptors with dopamine might lead to their down-regulation.

Resulting decrease in the amount of dopaminergic D2 receptors or just their sensitivity is unlikely to cause psychosis, similar to that seen in schizophrenia, but can make the person, for example, less able to be critical or filter the importance of incoming information. Results can range from increased creativity to suspiciousness.

Aripiprazole (Abilify) is another medication that is very effective as an adjunct to LDN and antidepressants for patients with decreased dopamine levels. Although this medication is officially classified as an antipsychotic, a class of medications that blocks dopamine receptors, it does not block them completely. Instead, aripiprazole keeps the receptors activated at a certain, steady level. For patients with elevated levels of dopamine, it leads to a relative decrease, but in patients with a low dopamine level, it leads to a relative increase in resulting activity. In some cases, this medication works wonders synergistically with LDN; in other cases, probably because of the relative increase in dopamine level, patients can tolerate only very small doses of naltrexone. Practice shows that aripiprazole is best used in conjunction with an antidepressant, not alone. One of the newest medications, Rexulti (brexpiprazole), is also a partial activator and partial blocker of dopaminergic receptors. Unlike Abilify (aripiprazole), it is more of a blocker than activator. Only time will show if its combination with LDN is more effective than with Abilify or Rexulti alone. Quetiapine (Seroquel) is another interesting example of a relatively safe antipsychotic that can improve serotonin-deficient as well as dopamine-deficient types of depression. Again, unlike other antipsychotics, it does not block the dopamine receptors completely. According to one hypothesis, it binds to the receptor and dissociates from it rapidly (the so-called "kiss and run" theory), providing not blockade, but just modulation of its activity.[33]

Providing building blocks for dopamine and trying to protect dopamine from depletion is another important strategy in LDN augmentation. This can be partially achieved by recommending certain foods—such as raw almonds, dark chocolate, bananas, apples, and strawberries; vitamins B6, C, E, and the antioxidants phenylalanine and tyrosine (up to 5,000 mg per day for a short time in severely depressed patients); and adoptogens such as *Rhodiola*, ginseng, and ashwagandha. Stress reduction and weight loss also help to preserve the supply of building blocks for dopamine.

Serotonin-Deficient Depression

While patients with a relative deficiency of dopamine crave stimulating foods such as caffeine or chocolate, patients with predominantly decreased levels of serotonin tend to crave dairy, bananas, and foods high in carbohydrates. Such depression is often accompanied by a lot of worrying and obsessiveness, as well as trouble sleeping. While dopamine-depleted patients reporting suicidal ideations often describe feeling that they have "nothing to live for," serotonin-depleted patients with depression, in contrast, report feeling suicidal because "life is full of pain and suffering." Normalizing serotonin levels can help eliminate these feelings, but will not necessarily make the patient feel happy. This is why LDN, with its dopaminergic effects, is important for them to take along with an antidepressant medication that acts predominantly on serotonin. On the other hand, attempts to alleviate depression with dopaminergic medications alone are less than spectacular.

Even if no serotonergic medication is used alongside LDN, we routinely recommend adding tryptophan or 5-HT, preferably with a small amount of carbohydrate and vitamin B3 or B-complex. Magnesium, zinc, SAMe (S-Adenosyl methionine), St. John's wort, and *Rhodiola* can also increase the level of serotonin.

Depression Related to Inflammation

Depression that is triggered by an inflammatory process is also likely to respond to LDN. Most people have inflammation of some sort, and exercise or stress can increase it. The stress hormone cortisol increases inflammation, and can also lead to the accumulation of body fat around the waist. Sometimes this alone, or, for example, discovering a small psoriatic patch that the patient did not think he needed to show to a psychiatrist, gives us a hint that a patient's treatment-resistant depression might respond better to LDN than to antidepressants. To enhance LDN's anti-inflammatory activity, our patients use St. John's wort (it is also a COX-1 inhibitor with an effect possibly greater than aspirin), willow bark, or arnica. We also prescribe omega-3 polyunsaturated fatty acids or their pharmaceutical forms such as Lovaza and Animi-3. There is an interesting product called Vayarol, which is a medical food made by combining krill oil with phytosterols. In addition to reduction in inflammation, Vayarol lowers triglycerides without elevation in plasma LDL-C levels.[34] Another example of a medical food that can be used along with LDN to reduce inflammation is L-methylfolate (for example, 15 mg or more of Deplin[35] per day). This works especially well for patients with increased body mass index. And finally, some examples of foods known to decrease inflammation include ginger, turmeric, pomegranate, green tea, and pineapple. Some changes in diet, such as avoiding processed food (including refined carbohydrates, sugar, fried foods, and processed meats); eating vegetables, fruit, and fish; and adhering to a modified Mediterranean diet can also help reduce inflammation.

Latest Research About LDN Use in Depression

Without good double-blind placebo-controlled studies, all theoretical reasoning remains as speculation and all practical experience is called anecdotal evidence. One of the latest research studies, "Low-Dose Naltrexone for Depression Relapse and Recurrence,"[36] conducted by David Mischoulon, MD, from Massachusetts General Hospital, was completed in June 2015, but no study results had been posted at the time of this chapter's writing. The purpose of this pilot study was to determine if taking a low dose of naltrexone (1 mg twice daily) in addition to an antidepressant medication could help treat relapse or recurrence in people with major depressive disorder. The investigators hypothesized that patients with breakthrough depression, on an antidepressant regimen containing a prodopaminergic agent assigned to treatment with LDN, would demonstrate higher rates of response compared to those patients taking placebo.

In my view, the researchers designed a very honest study. In the study, LDN was given to patients with a history of depression who already benefited from dopaminergic (the same action as LDN) antidepressants in the past but had relapsed into depression for four weeks prior to the study. To demonstrate that LDN is effective independently, beyond its dopaminergic effect, it was added to a dopaminergic agent, such as a stimulant, Abilify, or a high dose of Zoloft or Cymbalta (although Cymbalta is not a dopaminergic medication, it is believed to affect the dopaminergic transporter in the prefrontal cortex). Moreover, only the patients who did not respond to placebo were to be allowed into the maintenance phase of treatment. We anticipate that this study will be published soon and will provide objective evidence of the effectiveness of LDN in depression, confirming our practical experience.

– EIGHT –

Autism Spectrum Disorder

Brian D. Udell, MD FAAP

In the twenty-first century we are witnessing an epidemic of autism spectrum disorder (ASD), which the CDC now reports as occurring in one out of every sixty-eight children, and, alarmingly, one out of every forty-two boys.[1] The American Psychiatric Association's fifth edition of its *Diagnostic and Statistical Manual of Mental Disorders* (DSM-5) defines ASD as a condition that manifests in early childhood and interferes with normal development, in which affected individuals display persistent deficits in socialization and unusual repetitive interests or behaviors.[2]

The most challenging signs that patients exhibit are extremely aggressive behaviors and speech apraxia. Conventional treatment involves various therapies, such as applied behavioral analysis (ABA)[3] or speech and language therapy (S&L)[4] to address specific difficulties.[5] Indeed, a recent study revealed that six out of seven high-risk children who demonstrated red flags between the ages of seven and fifteen months returned to normal development by the age of thirty-six months under conventional treatment.[6]

However, conventional medical intervention involves pharmacologic preparations, including strong antipsychotics[7] and stimulants,[8] to dampen tantrums and aggression. Such medications are of questionable long-term value and carry a variety of serious side effects.[9] Furthermore, there is no listing in the *Physician's Desk Reference* of approved pharmacologic preparations that contains the words "speech apraxia." This situation is compounded by the additional central nervous system problems that ASD patients may suffer, about which modern medicine has little or no understanding regarding etiology or treatment, including:

- Fog: the appearance that the child exists in his or her own world, which is the very essence of the word "autism"
- Sensory processing issues: the over- or underfunction of sight, sound, smell, touch, and taste, which produces a variety of uncomfortable, unusual, and disruptive symptoms
- Cognition: expressive language lags far behind the receptive, which leads to unusual, unpredictable, or absent responses and the perception that there is lack of intellectual functioning

The myriad of signs and symptoms, combined with the paucity, lack of safety, and unreliability of conventional treatments, has led families to search for additional treatment options for their atypically developing child.

The goal of this chapter is to understand the spectrum of ASD, the role naltrexone has played in treatment so far, and how low dose naltrexone (LDN) is helping a variety of enigmatic conditions that present to a modern clinical practice in pediatric special needs.

Background about ASD

Prior to the 1960s, autism was thought to be the result of poor parenting. Dr. Leo Kanner, a staunch Freudian, first described it as a child psychiatric disorder in 1943.[10] Dr. Bruno Bettelheim, a mid-twentieth century media darling, amplified that misperception by ascribing ASD to the "refrigerator mom" theory of earlier days, which claimed that autism was caused by a lack of maternal warmth.

However, even as such misinformation was pervading popular and scientific thought, Dr. Bernard Rimland established the condition as a medical, not a psychiatric, disorder.[11] Among his many published works about ASD were an identification of fragile X syndrome[12] as a cause and vitamin B6 as a treatment,[13] a search for biomarkers[14] to identify the condition, and the unusual incidence of savants throughout the ASD population.[15]

By the 1970s Dr. Mary Coleman, a noted neurologist and author of *The Autistic Syndromes*, documented "an unusual exposure of parents to chemicals in the preconception period" in a series of seventy-eight autism patients. Twenty children were from families with chemical exposure; four were from families where both parents had such exposures: seven out of eight of those parents were chemists.[16] A similar report appeared in 1981, implicating external factors upon a susceptible population. "Eight of the

37 known parents of the autistic children had sustained occupational exposure to chemicals prior to conception; five were chemists and three worked in related fields. The exposed parents represented 21% of the autistic group. This compared to 2.7% of the retardation controls and 10% of the normal controls."[17]

By the beginning of the twenty-first century, two somewhat differing theories about ASD were beginning to take shape. Many resources were allocated to understanding genetic data, while some researchers, led by Dr. Martha Herbert,[18] offered a more holistic approach, proposing that ASD is "a whole-body disorder that affects the brain," rather than the other way around.

Presently, it appears that the combination of increased environmental toxicants acting on susceptible individuals is best treated by a biomedical approach to understand medical comorbidities, combined[19] with the traditional therapies of ABA, S&L, occupational therapy, and physical therapy.

Impact of ASD on Quality of Life and Morbidity

The diagnosis of ASD implies continued disability and the need for early and continued professional services. The goal of intervention is the mitigation of lifelong problems. Challenges are evident in early childhood by the lack of normal speech, leading to frustration and behavioral abnormalities. This often includes aggression against self or others, lack of socialization, and the requirement for specialized support. Extraordinary assistance is required throughout the school years, demanding treatments for medical and psychiatric signs and symptoms. The physical demands of resources and time and the financial constraints can become a huge burden. Parents' main concern is whether their child will ever be happy and productive. Finally, questions arise about how to handle patients who continue to have problems into adult life, where appropriate living facilities are scarce or out of ordinary reach.

In 1987, Dr. I. Lovaas reported:

> Follow-up data from an intensive, long-term experimental treatment group (n=19) showed that 47% achieved normal intellectual and educational functioning, with normal-range IQ scores and successful first grade performance in public schools. Another 40% were mildly retarded and assigned to special classes for the

language delayed, and only 10% were profoundly retarded and assigned to classes for the autistic/retarded. In contrast, only 2% of the control-group children (n=40) achieved normal educational and intellectual functioning; 45% were mildly retarded and placed in language-delayed classes, and 53% were severely retarded and placed in autistic/retarded classes.[20]

In 2010, Dr. Granpeesheh, "completed a study[21] which found that 6 out of 14 severely autistic children who obtained treatment by CARD had fully recovered." That's 43%.

A parent's discovery that their child exhibits developmental delays can create devastating effects on family dynamics. Extra resources must be allocated to the affected offspring, by way of time for services and therapies and extraordinary financial pressures allocated toward schooling and professional assistance. In 2014, the *Journal of the American Medical Association* published a study from the United States and United Kingdom that documented a cost for ASD of US $1.4 million over a lifetime, if there was no intellectual disability. That's $17,000 extra per child per year, representing half of the US median income. Add another $1 million if mental problems persisted (46% in one study).[22]

Even more alarming is the lack of experience with an emerging older ASD population. The literature on planning and existence of living facilities is sparse, so the ability to stave off the most debilitating signs and symptoms will have significant future effects.[23]

Current Pathophysiology of ASD

Multiple causes representing multiple pathologies have been implicated as producing the common signs and symptoms in children who fit criteria for ASD. Major[24] and minor[25] genetic alterations, infectious agents[26] and toxic agents,[27] atypical fetal development[28] and delivery,[29] mitochondrial and metabolic abnormalities,[30] and nutritional variations[31] have been implicated. Inflammation in the brain[32] and the gut[33] has been a consistent finding. The areas of the brain that are most implicated include the hypothalamus,[34] altered sympathetic–parasympathetic interaction,[35] and neurotransmitter differences.[36]

A common denominator in such a disparate group of possibilities is the presence of inflammation and oxidative stress, which leads to reduced energy production. Dr. Jill James has been reporting about the presence of impaired methylation since the beginning of this century. She has written that, "Relative to the control children, the children with autism had significantly lower baseline plasma concentrations of methionine, SAM, homocysteine, cystathionine, cysteine, and total glutathione and significantly higher concentrations of SAH, adenosine, and oxidized glutathione. This metabolic profile is consistent with impaired capacity for methylation (significantly lower ratio of SAM to SAH) and increased oxidative stress (significantly lower redox ratio of reduced glutathione to oxidized glutathione) in children with autism. The intervention trial was effective in normalizing the metabolic imbalance in the autistic children."[37]

Current Medical Therapy of ASD

Pharmacological interventions are usually aimed at the most obvious signs and symptoms of aggression, anxiety, repetitive behaviors, "stims" (also known as "stimming" or self-stimulatory activity, believed to be an expression of nonverbal communication), hyperactivity, and/or lack of focus including easy distractibility. There are few choices in each symptom category that are safe, effective, predictable, or on-label for children with ASD, which leads to a great deal of off-label use of psychogenic medications, such as the selective serotonin reuptake inhibitors (SSRIs),[38] which have only been studied in adult populations.

Biomedical intervention for ASD involves a thorough physical examination, review of systems, and laboratory testing to assess immune competence, inflammation, infectious organisms, vitamin and mineral deficiencies, gastrointestinal health, mitochondrial functioning, and energy efficiency. Successful treatment has followed a number of protocols that address specific issues with appropriate supplements, such as probiotics for gastrointestinal health,[39] food avoidance,[40] cysteine for oxidative stress,[41] carnitine,[42] and methyl B12 injections.[43] Often, parents report that homeopathic and naturopathic supplements[44] are helpful for specific complaints, which could be explained by their actions upon inflammation, energy production, and toxicity.

ASD and Naltrexone

Though naltrexone was initially proposed as an opiate blocker, as early as 1988 a study reported dose-specific reduction in self-injurious behaviors

(SIBs) in four autistic patients.[45] An accompanying paper measured beta-endorphin levels in forty patients with SIBs, and showed a positive correlation to unusual behaviors.[46]

The following year, tolerance to the medication was demonstrated in ten severely affected ASD children.[47] Behavioral improvements were noted as early as half an hour after taking naltrexone at regular doses, with improvements from verbal production to reduced stims. That led to a double-blind, placebo-controlled study of eighteen children, aged three to eight years, which yielded only mixed results.[48] A 1991 summary concluded, "The positive behavioral change seems to be enhanced by social support."[49] A safety and short-term efficacy study assessed forty-one children (ages three to eight), and again demonstrated mixed results.[50] As in the other papers, side effects were mild and transient in doses as high as 2.0 milligrams per kilogram (mg/kg).

A couple of years later, in a well-designed study of thirteen children (ages three to eight), eight subjects improved in two or more rating scales.[51] Another paper, while demonstrating only "modest clinical benefits," reported that the degree of improvement appeared to be related to the plasma chemical profiles, with significantly elevated beta-endorphins in all the children.[52] That suggested a subgroup with specific chemistries, "especially those related to the pro-opiomelanocortin system," would show the best response. Yet another article about twenty-three autistic children again showed mixed results.[53] In a study of twelve older autistic children (seven to fifteen years), seven improved.[54] "The behavioral improvement was accompanied by alterations in the distribution of the major lymphocyte subsets, with a significant increase of the T-helper-inducers (CD4+CD8-) and a significant reduction of the T-cytotoxic-suppressor (CD4-CD8+) resulting in a normalization of the CD4/CD8 ratio. . . . Changes in natural killer cells and activity were inversely related to plasma beta-endorphin levels." A replication study the following year reported "modest improvement of behavior in 11 of 24 children, but learning did not improve."[55] "No differences were found between the naltrexone (given for 2 weeks) and placebo conditions in any of the measures of children or parents' communication," in a 1999 evaluation.[56] Subsequent research in the early part of this century merely reiterated and synthesized those previous studies. The most common theme among the research at that time seemed to indicate that some patients responded to naltrexone with various and unpredictable improvements, from language, to hyperactivity and attention, to reduced irritability. Socialization behaviors, however, were rarely reported to improve.

ASD and LDN

In 2006, Dr. Jaquelyn McCandless reported on her informal, eight-week study of LDN on fifteen of her autistic patients, in which:

- Eight of the children had positive responses.
- Five of those eight had significant improvement.
- The primary positive responses involved mood regulation, cognition, language, and socialization.
- Two small children responded better when changed to 1.5 mg dosing.
- No allergic reactions were noted, and the primary negative side effect was insomnia and earlier awakening, usually fairly short-lived.

Dr. McCandless noted, "When LDN is given between 9 p.m. and midnight, the pituitary is alerted and the body attempts to overcome the opioid block with an endorphin elevation, staying elevated throughout the next 18 hours." Because of the bitterness of the naltrexone, it is applied as a cream while the child sleeps. Furthermore, she noted, "Although naltrexone is non-toxic and virtually free of side effects, occasionally it can cause sleep problems or hyperactivity during the first week or two of its use. If sleep problems persist, reducing the dose from 4.5mg to 3mg in adults, or in children from 3mg to 1.5–2mg, is often helpful."[57]

Further studies are needed to best identify individuals who are most likely to respond by increasing speech and communication, decreasing aggressive behaviors, and showing progress with social development, as well as markers (such as beta-endorphin levels) that reflect clinical improvement to enable better tailoring of the correct dose, and monitoring for side effects or toxicity.

Experience at a Pediatric Special Needs Clinic

There is no double-blind crossover, placebo-controlled, prospective research in this century that documents efficacy or patient selection of LDN for ASD. Safety is presumed due to the markedly decreased dosage compared to the previous well-designed studies. The following table is a

TABLE 8.1. Responses to LDN Treatment by ASD Patients

Response to LDN Treatment	Number of Patients (out of 53)
Significant Improvement	5
Satisfactory Results	19
No Improvement/Unsatisfactory Results	16
No Follow-Up Information Received	4
LDN Prescribed but Usage Not Initiated	9

chart review from a neighborhood clinic that specializes in developmental and special needs pediatric medicine. In 2014, fifty-three children (forty-six boys and seven girls, ages three to thirteen) with ASD were evaluated, treated with appropriate supplements and necessary medications, and prescribed LDN cream at a concentration of 3 mg per 0.5 cubic centimeter (cc). The increased concentration (vs. Dr. McCandless's protocol) has become preferable because the cream takes time to rub into the skin. These fifty-three patients were seen for a total of 393 visits (table 8.1).

Patients were selected as possible "responders" based on a number of factors, including history of repeated infections that interfered with developmental progress, aggressive or oppositional behaviors, and parental desire to avoid stimulant or antianxiety medications. One patient continued LDN treatment because their parent noted, "The child stopped getting sick all of the time." Significant improvement was determined by parents' observations that communication skills improved and/or that aggression was significantly reduced. Satisfactory results indicated that behavior improved enough so that the medication was reordered and utilized and behaviors seemed to abate. Most of the unsatisfactory results were because the parents saw no change, and only a few families became concerned about increased aggression, which was transient, lasting only a few days.

This protocol resulted in improvements noted in 45% of a selected population of the total population of high-risk infants and children who seek alternative treatments, because of the child's unresponsiveness to conventional therapy. This represents a significant improvement for many children who demonstrated immune system difficulties (repeated infections, unexplained fevers, high or low white blood cell counts, and out-of-range immunoglobulin levels) or negative behaviors.

Experience of a Selected Patient

Jacob, a three-year-old boy, was brought in by his parents after they were informed by a neurologist that their child had ASD, and the signs and symptoms were increasing.

His past medical history began in the first months, with significant sleep disturbances and incessant screaming diagnosed as gastroesophageal reflux, which required proton pump inhibitor medication. He continued to have extreme episodes of emesis, up to three times per day. By eighteen months, Jacob was not able to tolerate solid food. The mom was also concerned about the child's ability to breathe during these frightful episodes.

The diagnosis of speech delay was made at age two, at which time Jacob was showing other persistent, repetitive behaviors, such as staring, head banging, and running in circles. Sensory issues, such as the cry of his little sister or a toilet flushing, could set him off in a fit of punching and kicking. He eschewed human contact, even from his mom.

A thorough medical evaluation was begun. The physical exam revealed a well-developed, well-nourished, alert, awake, and oppositional hyperactive male who looked slightly pale, exhibited allergic "shiners," demonstrated low core muscle tone and delays in communication, with repetitive movements, and social isolation—all consistent with the diagnosis of ASD.

An initial protocol was started by appropriate, routine laboratory testing of blood, urine, and stool. Jacob was started on supplements targeted at improving gastrointestinal health and improving energy.

The parents reported that the earliest improvements were noted in increased speech and language. After the removal of gluten and casein, which tested positive in his allergy panel, new textures and foods were successfully introduced, and the vomiting ceased.

The aggressive behaviors continued, however, and the parents were reluctant to take the specialists' advice to administer Ritalin or Prozac, for example. They reluctantly agreed to administer Dr. McCandless's LDN protocol, applied as a cream, in the late evening.

Communication improved significantly thereafter, and the child was able to demonstrate his love and connection with the family and his mom. After more time and fine-tuning, he was able to return to a neurotypical classroom in a public school. In fact, Jacob is now somewhat famous for his newfound ability to play piano with ease!

Other Patients

The experiences of other ASD patients on LDN protocols may not be as dramatic, but are nonetheless impressive. Parents often report that their child wakes up happier, seems to concentrate and focus better, and gets along better in school. An apparently improved immune system leads some of the parents to exclaim, "I only give it 'cause he hasn't gotten sick in a year!" Indeed, all children regress a bit when they are ill, so these fragile patients seem to get benefit from this improvement alone.

Summary

Some doctors continue to prescribe traditional ASD regimens that continue to demonstrate improvement in patients, such as ABA. Some regimens wane in popularity, though they may reemerge, as in the case of secretin.[58] Others, such as Memantine, hang around until more testing is documented.[59] Unfortunately, many may cause harm, including Prozac and Zoloft.[60] A few are useful for specific purposes and so they continue to have a biomedical following. LDN treatment falls into this last category.

As in other conditions described in this book, gut dysbiosis involving small intestinal bacterial alterations is a common finding in patients with ASD.[61] Clinical practice reflects supporting research that improving gastrointestinal health is important in improving many of the most troubling signs and symptoms of ASD.[62] The utility of naltrexone to modulate immune responses may play an important role in effective treatment. Additionally, mast cell release of inflammatory chemicals such as IL-8 and TNF in the central nervous system has been implicated as a type of "brain allergy" in autism.[63] The finding that neurotensin, a mast cell-stimulating neuropeptide, is elevated in patients with ASD[64] is consistent with these observations.

Nearly two decades ago, Italian researchers wrote, "There is a growing body of evidence that the immune and the central nervous systems interact and reciprocally influence each other. . . . Taken together the assumptions that . . . the opioid system plays a crucial role in cognitive and immunological functions . . . and opioid peptides are present in excess in autism; then pharmacological reduction . . . by treatment with an opiate antagonist might counteract some of the behavioral and immunological disturbances observed in autistic individuals."[65] With a slightly different, low dose protocol, improvement was demonstrated "in a subpopulation of autistic children by chronic blockade of opioid receptors with a potent opioid antagonist, supporting the concept of an opioid-immune link in autism."

In clinical experience, there is a type of autism that clearly affects the patient's immune system. In such cases, parents complain that their children are sick all of the time; in other instances, allergic conditions such as eczema or asthma may complicate the clinical picture. Also, some oppositional behaviors are due to inappropriate coping mechanisms, similar perhaps to an externally chemically altered state, and appear to benefit from this intervention. However, there are a few major impediments preventing LDN from more common usage, including:

1. This condition is extremely complex. It is complicated by genetic and environmental influences and presents differently at different ages and even affects the sexes differently. Parents require information, resources, education, and support. With a myriad of presentations, response to various treatments will vary as well. Further research into how/why/who responds, and in what manner, is necessary.

2. The "spectrum" of autism needs to be better categorized and refined to take into account the various conditions that present with like symptoms, but are, perhaps, separate disorders.

3. No biomarkers exist to independently evaluate the extent of the problem and response to various treatment modalities.

4. Gastrointestinal health needs to be evaluated and properly addressed in order for improvement to be noticed.

5. After starting, the therapy requires continued tailoring to the patient's responses and the family situation. Some will have few resources and many other children, and so will tend to rely on conventional, available treatments as time and resources are at a greater premium. Other parents will utilize every available moment to search for answers to this enigmatic condition. Trying out new or unique treatments is within reach, though outcomes are quite variable.

6. Patients don't usually show immediate improvement; it may take up to eight weeks.

7. Not infrequently, an apparent deterioration in behavior may occur in the early stages of treatment.

It is important to note, of course, that many other biomedical interventions for ASD are subject to these same limitations.

Little has changed since 2006, when Dr. McCandless concluded, "As an effective, non-toxic, non-addicting, and inexpensive behavioral and immunomodulating intervention, LDN is joining our biomedical arsenal to help more and more children recover from autism as well as helping anyone with autoimmune diseases and cancer."[66]

LDN research involving an appropriate sample size; consistent product; duration of treatment; genetic, infectious, and metabolic information of "responders"; the effects of comorbidities; and the influence of other pharmacologic interventions will add a great deal to the successful treatment of this mysterious emerging childhood condition.

NINE

Cancer

DR. ANGUS G. DALGLEISH, MD, FRACP,
FRCP, FRCPATH, FMEDSCI,
WITH DR. WAI M. LIU, PHD

As of this book's publication, there have been only two controlled clinical trials on low dose naltrexone (LDN) and the treatment of cancer: one on breast cancer, which was terminated because of poor accrual, and one on glioma, which has finished but is yet to be reported on. Most of the clinical data with regard to cancer is therefore anecdotal or small series. A pioneer of the exploration of the use of LDN in treating numerous different conditions was Dr. Bihari, who as of March 2014 was reported as having treated 354 patients. According to the LDN website (http://www.lowdose naltrexone.com), he claimed an objective response of approximately 20% and stabilization in approximately 25%. If these were the results of a rigorous randomized trial, without other treatments, they would be most impressive, even by the standards of the newer, more active candidates of today. I was fortunate to visit the clinic once and to have read numerous anecdotes, but I felt at the time that the data included too many other co-treatments to justify the claims about LDN. However, in 2002 an oncologist and an assistant from the National Cancer Institute reviewed thirty charts from Dr. Bihari's office, of which half were chosen as appearing, without question, to have responded to LDN, confirming that there are several anecdotes where LDN appears to be the only major therapy that has led to clinical responses or long-term stabilization of the disease.

What is remarkable is that LDN's efficacy is not confined to any single tumor type, but involves melanoma, lung cancer, pancreatic cancer, renal cell cancer, prostate cancer, and lymphomas, among others.[1]

My own personal experience [AGD] with LDN treatment has included high-risk patients with multiple liver metastases who have failed standard chemotherapy, which has led to both long-term disease-free status and long-term stable disease. I also believe LDN has contributed to stabilization of aggressive disease in patients who have had tumor types other than melanoma, including advanced ovarian cancer and advanced prostate cancer. In addition, two patients who had both progressed through standard treatment for stage IV glioma had remarkable stabilization on LDN for six months, having progressed even during standard radiotherapy and chemotherapy.

However, it was the appearance of marked whole body vitiligo in a melanoma patient who started on LDN that raised the question of an alternative mode of action. He had progressed following a disease-free period of nearly four years, on an immunotherapy program given for nonresectable recurrence of a melanoma in the head and neck involving the neck lymph nodes. Upon recurrence of his pulmonary metastases, he was commenced on LDN and within one week developed severe whole body vitiligo, which is a feature consistent with activated cytotoxic T cells recognizing tyrosinase. This reaction was so powerful that I felt the LDN must have been operating through mechanisms other than opiate modulation. This led us to screen for new receptor interactions, which we describe later in the chapter.

Anti-cancer Properties of Naltrexone

It has been shown, mainly through the work of Dr. Zagon, that low doses of naltrexone are capable of suppressing tumor growth.[2] A definitive mechanism of action has yet to be established, but the effect could be achieved through direct antagonism of tumor growth or via modifications to the host immune system. Tumor outcome is a balance of growth and death, and naltrexone—as well as other opiates and opiate antagonists—is capable of altering this balance. In addition to their universally accepted analgesic qualities, opioids have also been reported to elicit a number of other cellular responses that lead to tumor death. The diversity of these effects has made it difficult to establish a major cause, and serves only to confound the identification of the principal mechanism of action. Indeed, they include those that are pro-survival in nature such as the induction of proliferation and protection against cell death, as well as polar opposite effects, including growth inhibition and the induction of apoptosis. The ultimate consequences of treatment with naltrexone are determined by dose and schedule. Nevertheless, studies exist to try to best delineate the action of the opioids and their cognate receptors, and in doing so design new therapeutic strategies to best utilize this fascinating class of compound.

In the early 1960s, it was reported that morphine possessed the capacity to disrupt the normal physiology of tumor-bearing rats.[3] The study was undertaken primarily to explore the appetite-disruptive nature of morphine on animals with tumors. However, in addition to showing that morphine could reduce the weights of these animals, the study also showed that tumor weights were concomitantly increased in those mice given morphine. The reason for this increase in tumor size was unclear, but it was perceivable that morphine could have secondary effects on the immune system, rendering the host more favorable to cancer growth. Indeed, morphine has been shown to be immunomodulatory in some instances, and thus it can alter the quality of the adaptive immune response.[4] Alternatively, the increase in tumor size could simply have been due to a direct effect of morphine that resulted in enhanced cellular proliferation or in reduced cell death. The induction of apoptosis is a biological necessity and forms parts of embryonic development and normal homeostasis, and as such, disruptions can lead to a variety of diseases and disorders.[5] Morphine has been shown to singly prevent both normal and desired cell death in the ciliary ganglion of the chick embryo, suggesting that in addition to modulating neurotransmission, morphine and other endogenous opiates may regulate neurophysiology.[6] In this case, the concentration of morphine appeared to be important, as apoptosis was only disrupted when used at higher doses; no effect was seen at lower doses. The importance of concentration was corroborated by another study, this time on rats, which showed higher morphine concentrations (25–200 micromolar [μM]) were able to protect primary rat neonatal astrocytes from apoptosis induced by nitric oxide.[7] In this study, it was also noted that the mechanism involved, in part, modulation of the PI3-kinase (PI3-K) cascade.

This opened the doors to the possibility that morphine and other opioids might be able to influence the growth and survival of cancer cells. This was indeed the case, and a number of review articles have summarized the influences that morphine has on tumor fate.[8] Unfortunately, the literature is still unclear and in many cases is contradictory. Reports simultaneously show that morphine is able to inhibit the growth of cancer cells as well as stimulate their growth in vitro. The cancer cells studied have been varied, representing virtually all cancer types, and all have been shown to be responsive. As some of these cancer cell lines express relatively low levels of the opioid receptors,[9] one suspects the effects may be both dependent and independent of these receptors. Furthermore, as both pro- and anti-cancer effects were seen in animal models, it has been postulated that the impact of morphine on the immune system is also likely to determine tumor fate.[10] However, the conclusions of a recent review added to the confusion by saying the evidence of an effect on anti-tumor immunity was inconclusive.[11] The effect of morphine on angiogenesis also cannot be discounted[12] and only reinforces the view that in addition to receptor-dependent mechanisms, opioids may influence cellular fate in other ways.

Opioid Receptors

Opioids exert their effects principally by binding and activating a family of G-protein-coupled receptors, of which there are many. The three main receptors—mu, delta, and kappa—share tight homology and can exist together to form receptor complexes. They also have their own specific patterns of distribution and can bind with a vast range of drugs and with differing affinities.[13] Binding to these receptors affects the action of the cell, and can, depending upon the ligand, stabilize the receptor complex, alter the stability of the states of other receptors, and affect cellular metabolism.[14] The opioid receptors are proteins that span the cell membrane and are coupled to a complex of guanine nucleotide binding proteins known as G proteins. Activation stimulates rearrangements of these G proteins, which ultimately lead to increased GTPase activity within the cell and stimulation of an intracellular response.[15] This response primarily disturbs the calcium and potassium channel function with the overall effect of disrupting Ca2+ movement and signaling via cAMP. Other responses include stimulation of members of the PI3-K superfamily via the actions of the released G proteins, which provides the entry into central-signaling pathways that modify cell fate. Furthermore, G-protein signaling is attenuated by a number of highly conserved receptor kinases that include beta-arrestin, which can phosphorylate and internalize the G-protein-coupled receptors (GPCRs), as a way of preventing tolerance by minimizing chronic stimulation.[16] Interestingly, beta-arrestins are also transducers of signaling, and the consequences of their action include activation of ERK+[17] and JNK,[18] which highlights another way that disrupting normal functioning of opioid receptors can activate intracellular signaling cascades. These activities also suggest new treatment combinations aimed at exploiting these observations.

Chronic administration of naltrexone increases the number of mu and delta receptors on cells.[19] However, the precise mechanism by which this occurs has yet to be defined. Evidence suggests that the up-regulation may be downstream of transcription[20] and independent of de novo synthesis of receptors molecules.[21] It is speculated that the increase in receptor sites to which a ligand can bind may be a redistribution of pre-existing receptors or from the increased recycling of the internalized form. Nevertheless, whether it is increased availability or increased sensitivity of the receptors, the increased numbers of receptors serve to enhance the interactions between opiate and opioid receptor.

Activation of the PI3-K and/or extracellular regulated kinase pathways through G proteins is not an effect unique to the opioid receptors, but most likely a generic feature of GPCR activation. This collateral effect possibly explains the anti-cancer effect of naltrexone and other opiates that is apparent via this secondary effect. One suspects that this is cell-type specific, which has only added to the confusion in the evidence that shows the effects of opiates can be both anti-cancer in nature as well as cancer-supporting. Furthermore, the manner in which the receptors are attenuated is different in each of the agonists,[22] and so the signaling cascade that is activated will also differ, leading to differences in the overall response. Thus for example, when morphine binds to receptors, it is in their agonistic conformation. This then elicits an intracellular response that chiefly works through alterations to Ca2+ currents leading to modification of synaptic functioning. Conversely, when naltrexone binds the same receptors, it is in their antagonistic conformation, and this then leads to a loss of receptor function through competitive inhibition, desensitization of receptor, activation of ancillary signaling systems, and initiation of cellular proliferation elements. Thus, for two drugs binding to the same receptor, the outcome is strikingly different.

Endorphins and the Opioid Growth Factor Receptor

In addition to the classic opioid receptors, there is evidence suggesting opiates are capable of eliciting response through other receptors. There is plasticity between the endogenous cannabinoid system and the opioid system; their receptors are members of the G-protein-coupled family, and they possess overlapping neuroanatomical distribution. There is evidence to suggest cross-communication of signaling pathways and activation of common physiological processes.[23] Indeed, the chronic administration of the cannabinoid receptor antagonist SR141716A can also modify the action of the opioid receptors.[24] Similarly, morphine can elicit a physiological response by cross-reacting with the somastatin receptor.[25] Taken together, it was postulated that exogenous opiates could modify the natural functions of other ligand-receptor systems in the body.

THE IMPORTANCE OF NALTREXONE DOSE IN CANCER ACTIVITY

In the 1980s, an in vivo study was conducted to explore the potential anti-cancer action of naltrexone. Mice were treated with increasing doses of naltrexone, and the main message of the study was that the dose of the antagonist was important in determining the overall effect. It was reported that, specifically for naltrexone, treatment in mice with clinically conventional doses (10 mg/kg) induced a continuous occupancy of the opioid receptors, which resulted in increased tumor growth.[26] However, if doses were reduced to 1 or 0.1 mg/kg, the receptor blockade was incomplete. Binding sites were thus available to exogenous opiates and endogenous endorphins, resulting in activation of their anti-tumor actions. Additionally, the schedule of administration was also crucial, with intermittent administration of lower concentrations of LDN achieving the greatest anti-tumor response. As reported previously, antagonism of the opioid receptors caused a compensatory increase in the amount of receptors available for binding. Thus, the short-term effect would be inhibition of growth caused by binding to the receptors of an endogenous ligand called the opioid growth factor (OGF); however, this benefit would be lost if naltrexone was left in culture. Thus continued presence of naltrexone serves to occupy new binding sites, rendering OGF unable to bind them, and thus no effect would be seen.[27]

Subsequent studies by the same group specifically exploring this growth modulatory effect of naltrexone also showed that the receptor associated with these effects, named the OGFr, was novel and significantly different from the classic mu-, delta-, and kappa-opioid receptors. Since this early work, much has been done to understand further the interactions between the OGF (chemically termed methionine enkephalin, or met-ENK) and its cognate OGFr, and their subsequent regulation of cellular growth and death.

Evidence for Activities Other Than through Opiate Receptors

Another observation that suggests that more than one pathway or activity may occur in vivo is the observation that LDN slowly improves some symptoms of multiple sclerosis, taking several weeks to manifest improvement, whereas some Crohn's patients report dramatic improvement within forty-eight hours of commencing LDN. Indeed, I [AGD] have witnessed such a response myself having commenced LDN in a Crohn's patient on steroids and anti-TNFα treatments who developed metastatic melanoma during this treatment. She was able to come off these treatments and remain solely on LDN for her Crohn's disease.

In view of these observations and the case of the patient with vitiligo mentioned earlier, my colleague Rachel Allen and I [AGD] decided to screen for other receptors, taking a very broad brush approach. We were delighted and somewhat surprised to find that naltrexone can greatly antagonize the TLR9 molecule. We were unable to confirm a report that it may use TLR4. TLR9 is exciting, as it is overexpressed in some tumors and many inflammatory states such as Crohn's disease.

Indeed, this may be the main mechanism that gives symptomatic benefit in Crohn's[28] disease, as it would explain the quick response. Both pancreatic cancer and glioma have had several anecdotal cases of benefit on commencing LDN. This work has been filed as a patent and will be published in the near future.

In order to establish whether LDN has specific effects at low doses as compared to higher doses, we [WML and AGD] have looked at the effect of exposing cell lines to different doses prior to looking at gene regulation. We are delighted to report that the genes that are up-regulated and over-expressed from normal when exposed to LDN are switched off, and that different genes are involved when exposed to higher doses. This work has also been filed and is the subject of another future paper.

Conclusions and the Future

There are many older drugs that have been reported as having new uses in the management of cancer. One of these is thalidomide and its successful analogues such as lenalidomide and pomalidomide. These analogues were developed in an attempt to enhance the known anti-TNF activity of thalidomide while trying to reduce major side effects such as neuropathy, which greatly limits the use of thalidomide in multiple myeloma, a condition that, surprisingly, improved with the addition of thalidomide with or without steroids. However, subsequent research has shown that these drugs enhance many other activities, such as being anti-inflammatory and co-stimulatory with regard to antigen presentation, in addition to being anti-angiogenic, all very desirable anti-cancer activities.

Other agents that have numerous effects on different pathways that may be beneficial in treating cancer include the cannabinoids, which have many features in common with LDN in as much as their effect on different receptors appears to be modulatory as opposed to agonistic or antagonistic alone. Indeed, there may be much to commend combining LDN and certain cannabinoid analogs in cancer treatment, although this requires further basic research.

There is a good scientific reason to take LDN seriously as having a potential role as an anti-cancer agent. First, it is an anti-inflammatory, a class of agents that have been proven to improve cancer outcomes as shown by numerous aspirin and COX-2 inhibitor studies as well as the surprising benefit reported with statins.

Second, LDN appears to have a marked immune modulatory response leading to an increase in innate immunity (such as natural killer cell activity) with a possible knock-on effect on CD8 adaptive T cells (the appearance of vitiligo after commencing LDN can only be explained by the induction of CD8 cells against tyrosinase).

Third, cancer patients can be suppressed by their disease, its treatments, and the psychological effects of living with a lethal condition. Patients report a remarkable benefit from commencing LDN with regard to their psychological status, feeling much better than on previous treatments, which may be due to its subtle effects on various opiate receptors.

Future research must focus on LDN's role as an additive agent with other treatments, as it can be added to most other treatments (with the exception of opiates) and, in the case of oncology, it appears to enhance the effects of some other treatments such as platinum. There is a very high chance that it will be most effective in some subtle combination. It is already sold with alpha lipoic acid and has been reported to be enhanced by the addition of metencephalin or OGF. However, the true benefit of these combinations remains to be shown in clinical trials.

Some combinations make perfect sense, such as making sure the recipient is vitamin D3 replete. Low vitamin D levels have been suggested as a major cause for nonresponse to LDN in multiple sclerosis patients, and low levels of vitamin D greatly reduce the efficacy of anti-tuberculosis chemotherapy and melanoma treatment. Mechanisms of action discussed previously strongly suggest benefit potential with immunotherapy such as vaccines, cytokines, and possibly checkpoint inhibitors. Similarities already mentioned suggest a great potential in combining LDN with the cannabinoids, to name but one example.

In summary, there are many reasons for developing LDN as an anti-cancer agent either as an adjuvant or in combination with other agents. Unfortunately, the numerous anecdotes currently reported still require confirmation with properly conducted clinical trials, which are very expensive. The cost of clinical trials is the major reason why they have not been done to date, as the intellectual property, based on current patent filings (over 350), is not strong enough to protect development.

It is hoped that this can be addressed in the near future and that LDN can achieve a license for adjuvant use in cancer management.

ACKNOWLEDGMENTS

One day last year, I received a message saying that Margo Baldwin from Chelsea Green Publishing wanted to speak with me regarding writing an LDN book. I thought, "What do I know about writing a book!" Needless to say, Margo was very persuasive, and I hope *The LDN Book* will be enjoyed by doctors and patients alike. I have to say there is far more work involved in having a book published than I realized. I naively thought when Gill Bell helped me gather all the articles for submission that my work was done! This wasn't the case; I have spent hours working alongside editor Michael Metivier, who was a pleasure to work with.

I would like to give praise to the late Dr. Bernard Bihari, who first used LDN in his clinical practice in 1985, as well as to the LDN work carried out in laboratories in the late 1970s by Dr. Ian S. Zagon and Dr. Patricia McLaughlin, and to the many doctors and researchers who have since followed in their footsteps.

Over the years it has been my honor to have worked alongside so many doctors, researchers, pharmacists, and other medical professionals who support LDN and the LDN Research Trust. I'm indebted to all our invaluable advisers, volunteers, and supporters, and to our patron, Jackie Young-Bihari.

A special thank you to all of the contributing authors and pharmacists for all their help with the book, Gill for helping put the chapters in the correct format, Michael for the editing, and Margo for trusting me to pull it off.

APPENDIX A

Starting the Conversation

Dr. Mark H. Mandel, PharmD

It's important to have good and valuable health-related information, but unfortunately, unless you can communicate that information to someone who can take action, it's a waste. First, you need to determine the appropriate audience to take it to. Then you need to know how to speak the appropriate language so that your audience can help you. The goal of this section is to give patients the proper tools to communicate information about LDN and its uses to decision-making practitioners, who can then use it to take productive action.

Sometimes, simply starting a conversation can be the most difficult part. Most of us are intimidated and reluctant to present our doctors with information because we don't feel we are fully equipped to do so. It is important to remember that as little as you may *think* you know about LDN, your audience will typically know even less. Therefore, in that initial conversation, you are the de facto expert. The responsibility of an expert is not necessarily to know absolutely everything there is to know about a topic, but to know what is pertinent to communicate at that time to that particular audience.

Reading this book, taking notes, focusing on those items that are most important to your specific condition, and organizing them in an outline or other structure that is easy for you to use as a communication tool are the first steps in communicating this valuable information to others.

When trying to communicate a new idea or message, it's important to keep the communication lines *free from static*. One of the most important aspects of this is to not make the recipient of the information "hang up" on you before you've delivered your message. There are things to avoid as well as things to focus on. When trying to get an unfamiliar message across to your health care practitioner (HCP), don't use words or terms such as:

- alternative medicine
- complementary medicine
- holistic approach
- natural medicine
- less dangerous approach
- miracle drug

These may be your thoughts or your motivation for wanting to use LDN, but they are terms that might be perceived as threatening or attacking to mainstream medical practitioners and could turn them off from listening to you further. Focus on the positive aspects of using LDN and not any of the negative aspects of conventional treatments unless you have had a personal negative reaction to a product that has previously been prescribed for you, in which case it is appropriate to bring up your specific clinical experience.

In today's information-rich environment it is difficult for HCPs to keep up with every bit of information on every topic. They have become accustomed to patients reading the primary literature on sources such as the National Library of Medicine (http://www.pubmed.gov), http://www.WebMD.com, or less-screened sources such as Wikipedia. Reliable websites such as http://www.ldnresearchtrust.org provide useful fact sheets that may be printed off and highlighted to provide the most important information that your HCP will need to feel comfortable writing your LDN prescription.

What practitioners are typically most interested in are:

- What are the potential benefits, and what are the potential risks?
- Will there be any interactions or contraindications with other medications or treatments that you, as the patient, are already using?
- How long will it typically take to see benefits from the LDN for your condition?
- What is the starting dose, and what is the typical progression to a therapeutic dose for your condition?
- What is the procedure if the optimal dose is exceeded and has to be diminished?
- Are there any lab tests that should be performed in advance of writing the LDN prescription?

As a patient, it is important that you become your most aggressive and knowledgeable advocate. HCPs have only a limited amount of time to see you, get the information that they need to make the decision to support your request, and act upon it. Do not simply print out the literature and hand it to your HCP. Read it before you go to your meeting and do your research so that you understand the data.

- Make the presentation simple.
- Use bullet points or a numbered list.
- Limit the bullet points to less than one page.
- Keep the information for your appointment brief and provide additional, more detailed information in a separate packet to hand to your HCP *after* he or she has heard what you have to say. If your HCP is distracted by your information too early, you can lose his or her attention.
- Index that information so that if your HCP chooses to read it, he or she can find the information readily.
- Pointedly ask your HCP if he or she has specific questions that you can answer when you have finished your presentation.
- Finish by asking your HCP if he or she will be writing the prescription today or if you should come back to the office tomorrow to pick up the prescription after he or she has had time to review the information in greater detail.

Practice your presentation in front of people you trust who will ask you follow-up and clarifying questions. Explain this role to your trial audience before you make the presentation, so that they know exactly what their job is. This will help you organize your presentation and will make it easier to present when it will be most meaningful.

When you make your presentation, you are essentially acting as a salesperson. In this case you are selling your well-considered reasons for wanting to try LDN. As the patient, you must ask for the prescription. Be firm but not pushy. This is your health. The HCP is there to take care of you and improve your health and your quality of life. If the answer is not affirmative and immediate then you must follow up and ask why he or she has not provided the prescription.

Set a specific follow-up time to communicate with your HCP. Ask about a preferred method of communication. For example, younger health professionals have told me that direct contact and phone calls are confrontational because they do not have a chance to consider their options of response.

They are concerned that they may not say exactly what they mean or in a manner that it will be received in the way that it is intended. They tend to prefer text messages, faxes, or e-mails.

HCPs have the same fears and discomforts that the rest of us have. It is important to not only use the proper words and terms but to provide them in a format that is conducive and comfortable for them.

Ask questions such as:

- Do you need more data?
- What data are you specifically looking for?
- What will make it easiest for you to feel comfortable writing the prescription?
- How would you like me to get you the additional information? (e.g.: fax, e-mail, hand delivered)
- How would you like me to contact you for follow-up?

Naltrexone is a very safe product in the doses that qualify as LDN. Naltrexone is FDA-approved and available commercially as an oral tablet in a 50 mg strength. It is approved as a treatment and deterrent for use in patients who are suffering from drug or alcohol addiction. The use of naltrexone in a low dose is called an off-label use. It is common for practitioners to use medications for purposes other than those that they are initially approved for. Examples of this include gabapentin, which is being used for pain management when it is FDA-approved for seizure disorders, and aspirin, which is being used for cardiovascular health or stroke when it was initially approved for pain and inflammation.

There are also many examples of medications being successfully used at doses other than the original approved doses or for purposes other than what they were originally indicated for. LDN is no different from these other medications in that respect.

This set of guidelines will hopefully make it easier for you to approach your HCP so that you can get the message across and can receive the care you need to improve your health and quality of life. Always remember that you must be your own greatest advocate, and if the practitioner you are working with is not sufficiently sympathetic to your needs, then it may be necessary to find someone more interested in your well-being.

Frequently Asked Questions about LDN

Skip Lenz, BPHARM, PHARMD, FASCP, FACVP,
with Julia Schopick, MA

I [SL] have been involved with low dose naltrexone (LDN) since 1999, when one of my multiple sclerosis (MS) patients asked if I knew anything about it. I didn't, so I started to look on the Internet, where I found a blog called *Goodshape*, which was run by a man named Fritz Bell. This was where I first became aware that MS patients were discussing LDN. There I found two names: Ian Zagon, PhD, and Dr. Bernard Bihari. I tried calling Dr. Zagon but was unable to get through or receive a call back. Dr. Bihari was busy, but his receptionist told me he would get back to me. And lo and behold, he did! This started a relationship that lasted until he stopped practicing medicine in 2007. Dr. Bihari was a gregarious, inquisitive, and friendly doctor who freely gave of his time to educate me. We had conversations about how LDN works, the conditions it works for, and his dreams for what he wanted to see happen in the future with regard to the drug. One of his mantras to me was to pass the information along, which I have tried to do, as have so many other people. I believe that he would be overjoyed at the success LDN has seen in the last ten years.

In honor of Dr. Bihari, I have made it my practice to answer any and all questions patients and doctors may have. You do not have to be a customer of Skip's Pharmacy to get some of my time. I have spent nearly every morning for fifteen years answering questions via e-mail, text messaging, and blogs. My afternoons are spent returning telephone calls about LDN. I started a compilation of these questions several years ago with the intention of writing a book. My book is on hold, but when Linda asked me to contribute a chapter to her book, I was delighted to have a forum to disseminate this information.

I have selected the twenty most frequently asked questions I get. I am presenting them here in the order of most frequency. I was surprised by some of the questions and hope that you find them—and my answers to them—illuminating.

Question 1: What do you use as a filler?

Low dose naltrexone, and all the drugs we compound at Skip's Pharmacy, may contain both active and inactive (or inert) ingredients. The inactive ingredients are called *excipients*. A filler is one example of an excipient. It is important that the fillers we decide to use interact well with the drugs we are using them with. Choosing the correct filler for a particular compound takes a great deal of experience.

To find the best fillers for LDN, I put together a team of pharmacists, pharmacy technicians, and pharmacy students and directed them to look at several fillers: calcium carbonate, sugar, microcrystalline cellulose (Avicel), lactose, and acidophilus. The team found that calcium carbonate was an inappropriate filler, but that the other four excipients dissolved quickly and freely. We ultimately chose sugar and microcrystalline cellulose as the most economical and easy-to-use excipients. However, in cases where the patient is diabetic or hypoglycemic, sugar is obviously not the filler of choice.

Many people have asked me why we decided not to use lactose or acidophilus as fillers. First, lactose is not particularly "compounding friendly" because the powders tend to fly around during the encapsulation process. Also, there are a very large number of patients who are lactose intolerant, so we chose not to introduce this as a contaminant into our compounding laboratory. Also, as I mentioned before, an excipient is an inert product. Acidophilus is an active ingredient. So unless the physician prescribes LDN specifically with acidophilus, we are compelled by state and federal statutes to use only inert excipients.

Question 2: I have (fill in the blank). Will LDN work for me?

I don't know how to answer this question when it is posed this way. A better question would be: "I have (Dx). Have you had any experience with using LDN for this diagnosis?"

Several years ago we conducted a survey of 1,173 MS patients who were taking LDN. We asked them four simple questions:

1. What is your diagnosis?
2. How long have you been on LDN?
3. Have you had an exacerbation or progression while on LDN?
4. How active was your disease prior to starting LDN?

We found that approximately 80% of our survey sample had not had an exacerbation or progression in over three years. Prior to starting LDN, the average patient had 1.3 exacerbations per year, so these results were very impressive.

We are currently looking at a new study group of 3,300 patients, all of whom are taking LDN. There is still a long way to go before the full survey has been completed. This time we added inflammatory bowel disease, chronic fatigue syndrome, arthritis, and other conditions to the survey. The results so far are extremely positive. Approximately 81% of the patients who are taking LDN have not had an exacerbation in greater than three years, and between 60% and 95% have had some relief of their symptoms. Again, impressive results.

Question 3: What are the side effects?

In our first survey approximately 8% of our patient population had some sort of sleep disturbance. The 81 patients who reported sleep disturbances resolved their issue in less than two weeks, and were able to continue on the drug with no untoward consequences. Only 1 patient was unable to continue. There was no other side effect that was experienced by more than 1% of the population. A quick scan of the current study suggests that side effect incidences are closely correlated to the diagnosis. We will have more information about the correlation in the near future.

Question 4: How long does LDN take to work?

Another badly worded question! First, you have to describe what you mean by "work." For instance, Dr. Bihari indicated that in his experience, "working" for MS patients meant that LDN would slow the progression of the disease or decrease the incidence of exacerbation. I created criteria for success for several other diseases for which LDN is used. For instance, for most of the other diseases, pain relief was one of the criteria. The success rate for the other diseases, which included rheumatoid arthritis, Crohn's disease, and fibromyalgia, was between 60% and 95%. In other words, 60% to 95% of patients experienced some relief of their symptoms.

On a personal note, I had juvenile onset rheumatoid arthritis (RA), and my pain resolved within three months after starting LDN. Subsequently we have seen an increase in the use of LDN for RA and have seen very good success. My impression is that it takes three to six months to get the same sort of pain relief that I have personally experienced with my RA. For other diseases, the amount of time is variable.

Question 5: I can't sleep. Why must I take LDN at bedtime?

The simple answer: You want LDN to be in your body and working during the period of time at which your endorphin levels are increasing naturally. This increase is coincidental with the dream cycle. It has been my experience that patients with an autoimmune disease do not generally dream very often. So when dreams come, the patient experiences them as "intense" or "vivid," and may cause them to wake up. Generally, this problem will resolve itself in a couple of days.

Question 6: Why do I need a prescription?

In the United States, LDN is a prescription drug. It is illegal to obtain a prescription drug without a prescription. In addition, you want your primary health care provider to know all of the drugs you are taking, so that he or she can better monitor your disease.

Question 7: Why doesn't my doctor know about LDN?

Naltrexone, in the commercially available dose of 50 mg, is a generic drug. It was approved by the FDA in 1984 for heroin addiction, and in 1994, for alcohol addiction. A generic drug is one that is not covered by a patent, and therefore a drug company takes some financial risk with producing it. There are no large manufacturers manufacturing naltrexone and therefore there are no drug salespeople or advertisements targeted at doctors to "educate" them about it. Doctors are creatures of habit. They will listen to the detail people and prescribe only those drugs that are produced by the big manufacturers. Without the protection of a patent, pharmaceutical companies will not go through all the necessary testing to have a drug approved.

Another problem is that doctors don't understand the mechanism of how LDN works, nor do they understand how high dose naltrexone works. As a matter of fact, most doctors don't understand anything about drugs that aren't used in their medical specialty.

Question 8: My doctor says LDN is a placebo. Is it?

I actually have a few answers to this question. First, there have been several studies done on using LDN for fibromyalgia, Crohn's disease, and MS. At the end of these studies there is always a caveat about how the results were positive but that further studies should be done. What this means is that the studies showed some good results but because the study population was not large enough, the results cannot be used definitively. The studies that doctors like to see are placebo-controlled, double-blinded studies, which cost in the region of several million to upward of a billion dollars to conduct. Therefore, most are conducted by large pharmaceutical companies. However, pharmaceutical companies are not about to conduct such studies on such a low-cost drug as LDN.

Our surveys, although not placebo-controlled or double-blinded, are powerful enough for me to be convinced that LDN works.

My second answer is rather snarky and begins with the question: "So what?" Personally, I don't care. I know that before taking LDN, I had major pain for most of my life. After taking LDN, I have been pain-free. Similarly, a majority of the thousands of patients I have spoken with and surveyed over the years have had similar results with LDN. I am quite sure they, too, would ask, "So what?"

Question 10: Can I take immunosuppressants with LDN?

This has been a problem. In the beginning, both Dr. Bihari and Dr. Bob Lawrence (UK) suggested that no immunosuppressants should be taken with LDN. Over the years this practice has been changed as a result of time and experience. Now I recommend that the short-term use of immunosuppressants is okay. As a matter of fact I recommend steroid bursts for MS exacerbations all the time.

Question 11: Can I take tramadol with LDN?

It should be well known that LDN cannot be taken with opiate pain medications such as oxycontin or morphine. However, I have long recommended that patients who must take pain medications consider tramadol, which is not an opiate, but works on similar receptors. The only problem can be with the amount of tramadol you take over a period of a day. Large amounts, that is, over 300 mg per day, have been reported to be problematic, but to my knowledge, lower doses (50 mg taken two or three times a day) have not presented any problems for patients while they are on LDN.

Question 12: Can I take LDN while pregnant?

Naltrexone 50 mg is classified by the FDA as a pregnancy risk category C, which means that there are no adequate and well-controlled studies in pregnant women. However, Dr. Phil Boyle, in Ireland, has told me that he has used LDN as an adjunct in his fertility practice for over ten years with no issues.

Question 13: My doctor said he cannot prescribe LDN.

What your doctor is saying is that he is not comfortable prescribing LDN, but he—and all doctors—*can* prescribe it. Off-label use of drugs is the practice of using a drug for an indication that has not yet received FDA approval. Every state in the United States allows for off-label use of drugs under certain conditions, as long as there is enough data to support its use. In the case of LDN, there certainly are enough small studies and enough "patient-based evidence" to support it.

Question 14: My doctor said that LDN is a narcotic and will not prescribe it.

LDN is not a narcotic. Your doctor is confusing narcotics with narcotic antagonists.

Question 15: Why does naltrexone have to be compounded?

The only commercially available product contains 50 mg of naltrexone. It is impossible for the layperson to divide these tablets accurately into the amounts generally considered for low dose naltrexone: that is, 1.5, 3, and 4.5 mg. Many patients attempt to do this, but I don't recommend it, especially when so many compounding pharmacists compound LDN so inexpensively and accurately.

Question 16: Why can't I just buy the 50 mg tablets from the Internet and make my own LDN?

This issue has been a longstanding point of contention. My short answer to this question is that you can't be sure of the quality of the 50 mg tablets you get online. In late 2014, I bought naltrexone from six different sites on the Internet. We had them assayed for potency. Not one of the six passed the United States Pharmacopeia standards. So yes, you can (illegally) obtain it through the mail at a discounted price, but like my pappy used to say, "You get what you pay for." In addition, please see my answer to Question 15 above.

Question 17: How much does LDN cost?

Each compounding pharmacy will set a specific price. That price includes the cost of the raw material, the cost of the compounding technician's and/or compounding pharmacist's time, and the associated cost of doing business.

Question 18: I am having an operation. How long should I be off LDN prior to the procedure?

Well, that depends. My first question is, "Has the doctor, dentist, or nurse told you which pre- and post-op meds you are going to be given?" The standard rule for opiates and for LDN is five times the half-life. Technically, this would mean that you could stop taking LDN as little as twenty hours prior to your surgery and be fine. However, I have known many people who have done just that, and some have not felt any analgesia and have experienced many of the side effects of opiates.

If the patient knows that they will not be receiving any opiates, I still suggest stopping LDN treatment seven days prior to surgery. Tramadol would be the analgesic I would recommend post-op. This will allow patients to resume their LDN fairly quickly. I always recommend that a patient confer with an LDN-knowledgeable pharmacist or physician prior to resuming their LDN.

Question 19: When should I take LDN?

We suggest taking it at bedtime.

Question 20: What dose should I take?

Some doctors recommend starting LDN at 3 or 4.5 mg. However, we recommend starting at 1.5 mg for thirty days. This is a very tiny dose, but it can still produce minor side effects. The second month, you should take 3 mg. This is a step up and should produce clinical results. Recently, after reviewing the literature and speaking with patients, we recommend that you stay at 3 mg for sixty days, see how you are doing, and then re-evaluate with your doctor to decide whether you should stay on 3 mg, or move to 4.5 mg.

Over the years there have been hundreds of different questions that I have answered on the phone, on the Internet, and in person. Most of these have been of a personal nature and do not apply to everyone, so I am not including them here. Some of my answers have been based on a patient's specific issues, which are not germane to anyone else. So if you have called and I have given you an answer different from one I've given here, it's because you are a unique individual and my response has been unique to you.

Finally, I would like to thank the worldwide family of LDN patients and advocates for letting me help you. The only way I have gathered the clinical knowledge I have of the use of this drug is by talking to you. Each and every one of you has had a hand in my education.

NOTES

Chapter One: The History and Pharmacology of LDN

1. M. P. Stapleton, "Sir James Black and Propranolol. The Role of the Basic Sciences in the History of Cardiovascular Pharmacology," *Texas Heart Institute Journal* 24, no. 4 (1997): 336–342.

2. M. D. Kertai et al., "A Combination of Statins and Beta-Blockers Is Independently Associated with a Reduction in the Incidence of Perioperative Mortality and Nonfatal Myocardial Infarction in Patients Undergoing Abdominal Aortic Aneurysm Surgery," *European Journal of Vascular and Endovascular Surgery* 28, no. 4 (October 2004), 343–352.

3. M. J. Brownstein, "A Brief History of Opiates, Opioid Peptides, and Opioid Receptors," *Proceedings of the National Academy of Sciences USA* 90 (June 1993): 5391–5393.

4. O. Schmiedeberg, *Über die Pharmaka in der Ilias und Odysse* (Strassburg: Karl J. Trübner, 1918), 1–29; and L. Lewin, *Phantastica* (New York, NY: Dutton, 1931).

5. Reginald L. Campbell and R. Everett Langford, *Substance Abuse in the Workplace* (Boca Raton, FL: Lewis Publishers, 1995); Brownstein, "A Brief History of Opiates."

6. Brownstein, "A Brief History of Opiates."

7. Campbell, *Substance Abuse in the Workplace.*

8. J. M. Scott, *The White Poppy: A History of Opium* (New York, NY: Funk & Wagnalls, 1969).

9. India: S. C. Dwarakanath, "Use of Opium and Cannabis in the Traditional Systems of Medicine in India," *Bulletin on Narcotics* 17, no. 1 (1965): 15–19. China: J. Fort, "Giver of Delight or Liberator of Sin: Drug Use and 'Addiction' in Asia," *Bulletin on Narcotics* 17, no. 3 (1965): 1–11.

10. Campbell, *Substance Abuse in the Workplace.*

11. Brownstein, "A Brief History of Opiates."

12. E. Hearne and M. C. Van Hout, "'Vintage Meds': A Netnographic Study of User Decision-Making, Home Preparation, and Consumptive Patterns of Laudanum," *Substance Use & Misuse* 50, no. 5 (April 2015): 598–608.

13. Ibid.

14. P. Prioreschi, "Medieval Anesthesia—The *spongia somnifera*," *Medical Hypotheses* 61, no. 2 (August 2003): 213–219.

15. G. Keil, "*Spongia somnifera*. Medieval Milestones on the Way to General and Local Anesthesia," *Anaesthesist* 38, no. 12 (December 1989): 643–648.

16. F. W. A. Sertürner, "Darstellung der Reinen Mohnsäure (Opiumsäure), Nebst Einer Chemischen Untersuchung des Opium," *J. Pharm. f. Artze. Apoth Chem.* 14 (1806): 47–93.

17. F. W. A. Sertürner, *Gilbert's Annalen der Physik* 25 (1817): 56–89.

18. D. Noble, "Claude Bernard, the First Systems Biologist, and the Future of Physiology," *Experimental Physiology* 93, no. 1 (January 1993): 16–26.

19. Ibid.

20. J. Sawynok, "The Therapeutic Use of Heroin: A Review of Pharmacological Literature," *Canadian Journal of Physiology and Pharmacology* 64, no. 1 (January 1986): 1–6.

21. M. C. Michel, "An Anthology from Naunyn-Schmiedeberg's Archives of Pharmacology," *Naunyn-Schmiedeberg's Archives of Pharmacology* 373, no. 2 (May 2006): 139.

22. C. C. Scott and K. K. Chen, "The Action of 1,1-diphenyl-1-(dimethylaminoiso-propyl)-butanone-2, a Potent Analgesic Agent," *The Journal of Pharmacology and Experimental Therapeutics* 87, no. 1 (May 1946): 63–71.

23. S. Hosztafi, T. Friedmann, and Z. Furst, "Structure-Activity Relationship of Synthetic and Semisynthetic Opioid Agonists and Antagonists," *Acta Pharmaceutica Hungarica* 63, no. 6 (November 1993): 335–349.

24. Sankyo Co., New morphinone and codeinone derivatives and process for preparing the same, GB Patent 939287 A, filed March 9, 1962, and issued October 9, 1963.

25. M. J. Lewenstein, Morphine derivative, US Patent 3254088, filed March 14, 1961, and issued May 31, 1966.

26. "Essential Medicines," World Health Organization, http://www.who.int/medicines/services/essmedicines_def/en/.

27. Endo Lab, 14-hidroxydihydronormorphinone Derivatives, filed December 6, 1966, and issued July 25, 1967.

28. C. B. Pert and S. H. Snyder, "Opiate Receptor: Demonstration in Nervous Tissue," *Science* 179, no. 4077 (March 1973): 1011–1014.

29. M. R. Hutchinson et al., "Evidence That Opioids May Have Toll-Like Receptor 4 and MD-2 Effects," *Brain, Behavior, and Immunity* 4, no. 1 (January 2010): 83–95.

30. M. Galanter and H. D. Kleber, *The American Psychiatric Publishing Textbook of Substance Abuse Treatment*, 4th ed. (American Psychiatric Publishing, Inc., April 2008).

31. K. Miotto et al., "Naltrexone and Dysphoria: Fact or Myth?," *The American Journal on Addictions* 11, no. 2 (Spring 2002): 151–160; E. R. Zaaijer et al., "Effect of Extended-Release Naltrexone on Striatal Dopamine Transporter Availability, Depression and Anhedonia in Heroin-Dependent Patients," *Psychopharmacology* 232, no. 14 (July 2015): 2597–2607; and "Naltrexone Hydrochloride 50 mg Film-Coated Tablets," medicines.org.uk, last updated March 5, 2014, https://www.medicines.org.uk/emc/medicine/25878.

32. J. E. Blalock and E. M. Smith, "A Complete Regulatory Loop between the Immune and Neuroendocrine Systems," *Federation Proceedings* 44, no. 1 (January 1985): 108–111.

33. Ibid.

34. Ibid.

35. B. Bihari, "Low Dose Naltrexone in the Treatment of HIV Infection," lowdose naltrexone.org, last modified September 1996, http://www.lowdosenaltrexone .org/ldn_hiv_1996.htm.

36. Ibid.

37. I. S. Zagon and P. J. McLaughlin, "Opioid Antagonist-Induced Modulation of Cerebral and Hippocampal Development: Histological and Morphometric Studies," *Brain Research* 393, no. 2 (August 1986): 233–246; and I. S. Zagon and P. J. McLaughlin, "Opioid Antagonist (Naltrexone) Modulation of Cerebellar Development: Histological and Morphometric Studies," *Journal of Neuroscience* 6, no. 5 (May 1986): 1424–1432.

38. R. N. Donahue et al., "The Opioid Growth Factor (OGF) and Low Dose Naltrexone (LDN) Suppress Human Ovarian Cancer Progression in Mice," *Gynecologic Oncology* 122, no. 2 (August 2011): 382–388.

39. S. Gupta et al., *Mechanisms of Lymphocyte Activation and Immune Regulation X: Innate Immunity (Advances in Experimental Medicine and Biology, Vol. 560* (New York, NY: Springer, 2005), 41–45.

40. Ibid.

41. C. Giuliani, "Nf-kB Transcription Factor: Role in the Pathogenesis of Inflammatory, Autoimmune, and Neoplastic Diseases and Therapy Implications," *Clinical Therapeutics* 152, no. 4 (July–August 2001): 249–253; and B. O'Sullivan et al., "NF-kappa B as a Therapeutic Target in Autoimmune Disease," *Expert Opinion on Therapeutic Topics* 11, no. 2 (February 2007): 111–122.

42. C. S. Mitsiades, "Activation of NF-kappa B and Upregulation of Intracellular Anti-Apoptotic Proteins via the IGF-1/Akt Signalling in Human Multiple Myeloma Cells: Therapeutic Implications," *Oncogene* 21, no. 37 (August 2002): 5673–5683.

43. M. R. Hutchinson et al, "Non-Stereoselective Reversal of Neuropathic Pain by Naloxone and Naltrexone: Involvement of Toll-Like Receptor 4 (TLR4)," *European Journal of Neuroscience* 28, no. 1 (July 2008): 20–29.

44. Ibid.

45. Ibid.

46. A. Marshak-Rothstein, "Toll-Like Receptors in Systemic Autoimmune Disease," *Nature Reviews Immunology* 6, no. 11 (November 2006): 823–835; V. D. Pradhan et al., "Toll-Like Receptors in Autoimmunity with Special Reference to Systemic Lupus Erythematosus," *Indian Journal of Human Genetics* 18, no. 2 (May–August 2012): 155–160; A. Marshak-Rothstein, "Toll-Like Receptors in Systemic Autoimmune Disease," *Nature Reviews Immunology* 6, no. 11 (November 2006): 823–835; and D. Singh and S. Naik, "The Role of Toll-Like Receptors in Autoimmune Diseases," *Journal of Indian Rheumatology Association* 13 (2005): 162–165.

47. L. A. J. O'Neill, "Toll-Like Receptors in Cancer," *Oncogene* 27 (2008): 158–160.

Chapter Two: Multiple Sclerosis and Lupus

1. C. Lucchinetti et al., "Heterogeneity of Multiple Sclerosis Lesions: Implications for the Pathogenesis of Demyelination," *Annals of Neurology* 47, no. 6 (June 2000): 707–717.

2. A. Minagar et al., "Multiple Sclerosis as a Vascular Disease," *Neurological Research* 28, no. 3 (April 2006): 230–235.

3. B. Ferreira et al., "Glutathione in Multiple Sclerosis," *British Journal of Biomedical Science* 70, no. 2 (2013): 75–79; A. Hadzovic-Dzuvo et al., "Serum Total Antioxidant Capacity in Patients with Multiple Sclerosis," *Bosnian Journal of Basic Medical Sciences* 11, no. 1 (February 2011): 33–36; G. G. Ortiz et al, "Oxidative Stress Is Increased in Serum from Mexican Patients with Relapsing-Remitting Multiple Sclerosis," *Disease Markers* 26, no. 1 (2009): 35–39; E. Miller et al., "Oxidative Stress in Multiple Sclerosis," *Polski Merkuriusz Lekarski* 27, no. 162 (December 2009): 499–502; J. Van Horssen et al., "Radical Changes in Multiple Sclerosis Pathogenesis," *Biochimica et Biophysica Acta* 1812, no. 2 (February 2011): 141–150; M. T. Lin and M. Flint Beal, "Review Article Mitochondrial Dysfunction and Oxidative Stress in Neurodegenerative Diseases," *Nature* 443 (October 2006): 787–795; and R. Srinivasan et al., "MR Spectroscopic Imaging of Glutathione in the White and Gray Matter at 7 T with an Application to Multiple Sclerosis," *Magnetic Resonance Imaging* 28, no. 2 (February 2010): 163–170.

4. A. Compton and A. Coles, "Multiple Sclerosis," *The Lancet Seminars: The Lancet Core Clinical Collection* 372, no. 9648 (October 2008): 1502–1571.

5. R. Voskuhl, *MS Connection Blog*, February 14, 2014.

6. J. L. Huynh and P. Casaccia, "Epigenetic Mechanisms in Multiple Sclerosis: Implications for Pathogenesis and Treatment," *The Lancet Neurology* 12, no. 2 (February 2013): 195–206.

7. Ibid.

8. B. Richardson, "Primer: Epigenetics of Autoimmunity," *Natural Clinical Practice Rheumatology* 3, no. 9 (September 2007): 521–527.

9. M. Trivedi et al., "Morphine Induces Redox-Based Changes in Global DNA Methylation and Retrotransposon Transcription by Inhibition of Excitatory Amino Acid Transporter Type 3–Mediated Cysteine Uptake," *Molecular Pharmacology* 85, no. 5 (May 2014): 747–757.

10. B. Locwin, "How Epigenetics, Our Gut Microbiome and the Environment Interact to Change Our Lives," *Genetic Literacy Project*, September 15, 2014, http://www.geneticliteracyproject.org/2014/09/15/how-epigenetics-our-gut-microbiome-and-the-environment-interact-to-change-our-lives/#link.

11. F. P. Perera, "Molecular Epidemiology: Insights into Cancer Susceptibility, Risk Assessment, and Prevention," *Journal of the National Cancer Institute* 88, no. 8 (April 1996): 496–509.

12. Lucchinetti et al., "Heterogeneity of Multiple Sclerosis Lesions."

13. J. M. Ridlon et al., "*Clostridium scindens*: A Human Gut Microbe with a High Potential to Convert Glucocorticoids into Androgens," *The Journal of Lipid Research* 54, no. 9 (September 2013): 2437–2449.

14. K. O'Rourke, "Study Hints Gut Microbiome Plays a Role in Multiple Sclerosis," *Gastroenterology & Endoscopy News*, December 2014, http://www.gastroendo news.com/ViewArticle.aspx?d=In+the+News&d_id=187&i=December+2014&i _id=1133&a_id=28944.

15. R. Gandhi et al., "Gut Microbiome Is Linked to Immune Cell Phenotype in Multiple Sclerosis," *Joint ACTRIMS-ECTRIMS Meeting* (2014) P616.

16. B. Stetka, "Could Multiple Sclerosis Begin in the Gut?," *Scientific American*, October 8, 2014, http://www.scientificamerican.com/article/could-multiple-sclerosis-begin-in-the-gut/; and P. Bhargava and E. M. Mowry, "Gut Microbiome and Multiple Sclerosis," *Current Neurology and Neuroscience Reports* 14, no. 10 (October 2014): 492.

17. S. M. Vieira et al., "Diet, Microbiota and Autoimmune Diseases," *Lupus* 23, no. 6 (May 2014): 518–526.

18. Ibid.

19. F. Lutgendorff et al., "The Role of Microbiota and Probiotics in Stress-Induced Gastro-Intestinal Damage," *Current Molecular Medicine* 8, no. 4 (June 2008): 282–298.

20. "Diet Affects Men's and Women's Gut Microbes Differently," *UTNews*, July 29, 2014, http://news.utexas.edu/2014/07/29/diet-affects-microbes -differently-by-gender; and Anita Chhabra et al., "A Role for Hormones, Gut Microbiota and Tolerogenic CD103DC in Protection of Male (NZBxNZW)F1 (BWF1) Mice from Lupus (MUC8P.805)," *The Journal of Immunology* 192 (May 2014).

21. S. M. Snedeker and A. G. Hay, "Do Interactions between Gut Ecology and Environmental Chemicals Contribute to Obesity and Diabetes?," *Environmental Health Perspectives* 120, no. 3 (March 2012): 332–339; and A. Samsel and S. Seneff, "Glyphosate's Suppression of Cytochrome P450 Enzymes and Amino Acid Biosynthesis by the Gut," *Entropy* 15, no. 4 (2013): 1416–1463.

22. M. Hadjivassiliou et al., "Gluten Sensitivity as a Neurological Illness," *Journal of Neurology, Neurosurgery, & Psychiatry* 72, no. 5 (May 2002): 560–563.

23. M. S. Trivedi et al., "Food-Derived Opioid Peptides Inhibit Cysteine Uptake with Redox and Epigenetic Consequences," *Journal of Nutritional Biochemistry* 25, no. 10 (October 2014): 1011–1018.

24. David Perlmutter, *Grain Brain* (New York, NY: Little, Brown and Company, 2013), 58–60.

25. Ibid.

26. T. Suzuki et al., "Low Serum Levels of Dehydroepiandrosterone May Cause Deficient IL-2 Production by Lymphocytes in Patients with Systemic Lupus Erythematosus (SLE)," *Clinical & Experimental Immunology* 99, no. 2 (February 1995): 251–255.

27. Perlmutter, *Grain Brain*, 58.

28. A. Fasano, "Zonulin and Its Regulation of Intestinal Barrier Function: The Biological Door to Inflammation, Autoimmunity, and Cancer," *Physiological Reviews* 91, no. 1 (January 2011): 151–175.

29. R. L. Swank, "Multiple Sclerosis: Fat-Oil Relationship," *Nutrition* 7, no. 5 (September–October 1991): 368–376.

30. K. Takata et al., "Intestinal Microflora Modified by *Candida kefyr* Reduces the Susceptibility to Experimental Autoimmune Encephalomyelitis," *Annals of Clinical and Translational Neurology* 2, no. 1 (January 2015): 56–66.

31. M. J. Glass et al., "Naltrexone Administered to Central Nucleus of Amygdala or PVN: Neural Dissociation of Diet and Energy," *American Journal of Physiology: Regulatory, Integrative and Comparative Physiology* 279, no. 1 (July 2000): R86–92; Ashley E. Mason et al., "Putting the Brakes on the Drive to Eat: Pilot Effects of Naltrexone and Reward-Based Eating on Food Cravings among Obese Women," *Eating Behaviors* 19 (December 2015): 53–56; and M. R. Yeomans and R. W. Gray, "Effects of Naltrexone on Food Intake and Changes of Subjective Appetite during Eating: Evidence of Opioid Involvement in the Appetizer Effect," *Physiology & Behavior* 62, no. 1 (July 1997): 15–21.

32. J. A. Majde and J. M. Krueger, "Links between the Innate Immune System and Sleep," *Journal of Allergy and Clinical Immunology* 116, no. 6 (December 2005): 1188–1198.

33. A. Falini et al., "Differential Diagnosis of Posterior Fossa Multiple Sclerosis Lesions—Neuroradiological Aspects," *Neurological Sciences* 22 (November 2001): S79–83.

34. J. Chmielewska-Badora et al., "Lyme Borreliosis and Multiple Sclerosis: Any Connection?," *Annals of Agricultural and Environmental Medicine* 7, no. 2 (2000): 141–143.

35. M. Fritzsche, "Chronic Lyme Borreliosis at the Root of Multiple Sclerosis—Is a Cure with Antibiotics Attainable?," *Medical Hypotheses* 64, no. 3 (2005): 438–448.

36. A. Maxmen, "Antibodies Linked to Long-Term Lyme Symptoms," *Nature*, August 5, 2011, http://www.nature.com/news/2011/110805/full/news.2011.463.html.

37. E. Kassi and P. Moutsatsou, "Estrogen Receptor Signaling and Its Relationship to Cytokines in Systemic Lupus Erythematosus," *Journal of Biomedicine and Biotechnology* (2010); and V. Tomassini et al., "Sex Hormones Modulate Brain Damage in Multiple Sclerosis: MRI Evidence," *Journal of Neurology, Neurosurgery, and Psychiatry* 76, no. 2 (February 2005): 272–275.

38. A. Carrillo-Vico et al., "Melatonin: Buffering the Immune System," *International Journal of Molecular Sciences* 14, no. 4 (April 2013): 8638–8683.

39. S. A. Ahmed, "The Immune System as a Potential Target for Environmental Estrogens (Endocrine Disrupters): A New Emerging Field," *Toxicology* 150, nos. 1–3 (September 2000): 191–206; and B. Jung and N. Ahmad, "Melatonin in Cancer Management: Progress and Promise," *Cancer Research* 66, no. 20 (October 2006): 9789–9793.

40. R. A. McKinnon and D. W. Nebert, "Possible Role of Cytochromes P450 in Lupus Erythematosus and Related Disorders," *Lupus* 3, no. 6 (December 1994): 473–478.

41. L. Korkina et al., "The Chemical Defensive System in the Pathobiology of Idiopathic Environment-Associated Diseases," *Current Drug Metabolism* 10, no. 8 (October 2009): 914–931.

42. D. J. Nakazawa, *The Autoimmune Epidemic* (New York, NY: Touchstone, 2009).

43. L. H. Burns, "Ultra-Low-Dose Opioid Antagonists Enhance Opioid Analgesia while Reducing Tolerance, Dependence and Addictive Properties. Recent Developments in Pain Research," *Recent Developments in Pain Research* (2005): 115–136.

44. C. Pierrot-Deseilligny, "Clinical Implications of a Possible Role of Vitamin D in Multiple Sclerosis," *Journal of Neurology* 256, no. 9 (September 2009): 1468–1479.

45. S. M. Kimball et al., "Safety of Vitamin D3 in Adults with Multiple Sclerosis," *American Journal of Clinical Nutrition* 86, no. 3 (September 2007): 645–651.

46. J. M. Burton et al., "A Phase I/II Dose-Escalation Trial of Vitamin D3 and Calcium in Multiple Sclerosis," *Neurology* 74, no. 23 (June 2010): 1852–1859.

47. Y. Arnson et al., "Vitamin D and Autoimmunity: New Aetiological and Therapeutic Considerations," *Annals of the Rheumatic Diseases* 66, no. 9 (September 2007): 1137–1142.

48. "Vitamin D Linked to Autoimmune and Cancer Disease Genes, Underscoring Risks of Deficiency," *U.S. News Health*, August 24, 2010, http://health.usnews.com /health-news/diet-fitness/diabetes/articles/2010/08/24/vitamin-d-may-influence -genes-for-cancer-autoimmune-disease.

49. S. V. Ramagopalan et al., "A ChIP-seq-Defined Genome-Wide Map of Vitamin D Receptor Binding: Associations with Disease and Evolution," *Genome Research* 20, no. 10 (October 2010): 1352–1360.

50. Arnson et al., "Vitamin D and Autoimmunity."

51. L. Dehghani et al., "Can Vitamin D Suppress Endothelial Cells Apoptosis in Multiple Sclerosis Patients?," *International Journal of Preventative Medicine* 4 (May 2013): S211–215.

52. A. N. Carvalho et al., "Glutathione in Multiple Sclerosis: More Than Just an Antioxidant?," *Multiple Sclerosis* 20, no. 11 (October 2014): 1425–1431.

53. L. Packer et al., "Neuroprotection by the Metabolic Antioxidant α-Lipoic Acid," *Free Radical Biology & Medicine* 22, nos. 1–2 (1997): 359–378.

54. G. H. Marracci et al., "Alpha Lipoic Acid Inhibits T Cell Migration into the Spinal Cord and Suppresses and Treats Experimental Autoimmune Encephalomyelitis," *Journal of Neuroimmunology* 131, nos. 1–2 (October 2002): 104–114; and G. Schreibelt et al., "Lipoic Acid Affects Cellular Migration into the Central Nervous System and Stabilizes Blood-Brain Barrier Integrity," *Journal of Immunology* 177, no. 4 (August 2006): 2630–2637.

55. Hadzovic-Dzuvo et al., "Serum Total Antioxidant Capacity."

56. M. E. van Meeteren et al., "Antioxidants and Polyunsaturated Fatty Acids in Multiple Sclerosis," *European Journal of Clinical Nutrition* 59, no. 12 (December 2005): 1347–1361.

57. F. Sedel, "High Doses of Biotin in Chronic Progressive Multiple Sclerosis: A Pilot Study," *Multiple Sclerosis and Related Disorders* 4, no. 2 (March 2015): 159–169.

58. Carrillo-Vico et al., "Melatonin: Buffering the Immune System."

59. Jung and Ahmad, "Melatonin in Cancer Management."

60. P. Mao et al., "MitoQ, a Mitochondria-Targeted Antioxidant, Delays Disease Progression and Alleviates Pathogenesis in an Experimental Autoimmune Encephalomyelitis Mouse Model of Multiple Sclerosis," *Biochimica Biophysica Acta* 1832, no. 12 (December 2013): 2322–2331.

61. S. M. Toloza et al., "Vitamin D Insufficiency in a Large Female SLE Cohort," *Lupus* 19, no. 1 (January 2010): 13–19.

62. Ramagopalan et al., "A ChIP-seq-Defined Genome-Wide Map."

63. C. C. Mok et al., "Vitamin D Deficiency as Marker for Disease Activity and Damage in Systemic Lupus Erythematosus: A Comparison with Anti-dsDNA and Anti-C1q," *Lupus* 21, no. 1 (January 2012): 36–42.

64. Arnson et al., "Vitamin D and Autoimmunity."

65. D. Bruce et al., "Converging Pathways Lead to Overproduction of IL-17 in the Absence of Vitamin D Signaling," *International Immunology* 23, no. 8 (August 2011): 519–528.

66. B. Terrier et al., "Restoration of Regulatory and Effector T Cell Balance and B Cell Homeostasis in Systemic Lupus Erythematosus Patients through Vitamin D Supplementation," *Arthritis Research & Therapy* 14, no. 5 (October 2012): R221.

67. S. A. Rogers, *Detoxify or Die* (Sovay, NY: Prestige Publishing, 2002).

68. "Body Burden: The Pollution in Newborns. A Benchmark Investigation of Industrial Chemicals, Pollutants and Pesticides in Umbilical Cord Blood," *EWG*, July 14, 2005, http://www.ewg.org/research/body-burden-pollution-newborns.

69. "The Most Poorly Tested Chemicals in the World," *Chemical Industry Archives*, March 27, 2009, http://www.chemicalindustryarchives.org/factfiction/testing.asp.

70. D. J. Nazawaka, *The Automimmune Epidemic* (New York, NY: Touchstone, 2008), 89–123.

71. L. Balluz et al., "Investigation of Systemic Lupus Erythematosus in Nogales, Arizona," *American Journal of Epidemiology* 154, no. 11 (December 2001): 1029–1036.

72. R. W. McMurray and W. May, "Sex Hormones and Systemic Lupus Erythematosus: Review and Meta-Analysis," *Arthritis & Rheumatology* 48, no. 8 (August 2003): 2100–2110.

73. S. Appenzeller et al., "Prevalence of Thyroid Dysfunction in Systemic Lupus Erythematosus," *Journal of Clinical Rheumatology* 15, no. 3 (April 2009): 117–119.

74. Stetka, "Could Multiple Sclerosis Begin in the Gut?"; Dehghani et al., "Can Vitamin D Suppress Endothelial Cells Apoptosis"; N. Tellez et al., "Fatigue in Progressive Multiple Sclerosis Is Associated with Low Levels of Dehydroepiandrosterone," *Multiple Sclerosis* 12, no. 4 (August 2006): 487–494; F. Kapsimalis et al., "Cytokines and Normal Sleep," *Current Opinion in Pulmonary Medicine* 11, no. 6 (November 2005): 481–484; A. T. Y. Chan et al., "Thyroid Disease in Systemic Lupus Erythematosus and Rheumatoid Arthritis," *Rheumatology* 40, no. 3 (2001): 353–354; and Korkina et al., "The Chemical Defensive System."

75. "Disease Clusters Spotlight the Need to Protect People from Toxic Chemicals," *Natural Resources Defense Council*, May 10, 2011, http://www.nrdc.org/health/diseaseclusters/.

76. J. J. Powell, "Evidence for the Role of Environmental Agents in the Initiation or Progression of Autoimmune Conditions," *Environmental Health Perspectives* 107, no. 5 (October 1999): 667–672.

77. N. Ballatori, "Transport of Toxic Metals by Molecular Mimicry," *Environmental Health Perspectives* 110, no. 5 (October 2002): 689–694.

78. Rogers, *Detoxify or Die*; and Ahmed, "The Immune System as a Potential Target."

79. *Genetic Roulette: The Gamble of Our Lives*, directed by Jeffrey M. Smith (Institute for Responsible Technology, 2012), Film.

80. Richardson, "Primer: Epigenetics of Autoimmunity."

81. P. Sarzi-Puttini et al., "Environment and Systemic Lupus Erythematosus: An Overview," *Autoimmunity* 38, no. 7 (November 2005): 465–472.

82. M. D. Mayes, "Epidemiologic Studies of Environmental Agents and Systemic Autoimmune Diseases," *Environmental Health Perspectives* 107, no. 5 (October 1999): 743–748.

83. P. B. Tchounwou et al., "Review: Environmental Exposure to Mercury and Its Toxicopathologic Implications for Public Health," *Environmental Toxicology* 18, no. 3 (June 2003): 149–175.

84. Ballatori, "Transport of Toxic Metals."

85. Srinivasan et al., "MR Spectroscopic Imaging of Glutathione."

86. Ferreira et al., "Glutathione in Multiple Sclerosis"; Hadzovic-Dzuvo et al., "Serum Total Antioxidant Capacity in Patients"; Ortiz et al., "Oxidative Stress Is Increased"; Miller et al., "Oxidative Stress in Multiple Sclerosis"; van Horssen et al., "Radical Changes in Multiple Sclerosis Pathogenesis"; Lin and Beal, "Review Article Mitochondrial Dysfunction"; and Srinivasan et al., "MR Spectroscopic Imaging of Glutathione."

87. Mckinnon and Nebert, "Possible Role of Cytochromes P450."

88. L. Korkina et al., "The Chemical Defensive System in the Pathobiology of Idiopathic Environment-Associated Diseases," *Current Drug Metabolism* 10, no. 8 (October 2009): 914–931.

89. Samsel and Seneff, "Glyphosate's Suppression of Cytochrome P450."

90. Nazawaka, *The Autoimmune Epidemic*.

91. Trivedi et al., 2014.

92. Kassi and Moutsatsou, "Estrogen Receptor Signaling"; and C.M. Grimaldi, "Sex and Systemic Lupus Erythematosus: The Role of the Sex Hormones Estrogen and Prolactin on the Regulation of Autoreactive B Cells," *Current Opinion in Rheumatology* 18, no. 5 (September 2006): 456–461.

93. Kassi and Moutsatsou, "Estrogen Receptor Signaling."

94. Ahmed, "The Immune System as a Potential Target."

95. M. Kipp et al., "Multiple Sclerosis: Neuroprotective Alliance of Estrogen–Progesterone and Gender," *Frontiers in Neuroendocrinology* 33, no. 1 (January 2012): 1–16.

96. K. Lelu et al., "Estrogen Receptor α Signaling in T Lymphocytes Is Required for Estradiol-Mediated Inhibition of Th1 and Th17 Cell Differentiation and

Protection against Experimental Autoimmune Encephalomyelitis," *The Journal of Immunology* 187, no. 5 (September 2011): 2386–2393.

97. S. S. Soldan, "Immune Modulation in Multiple Sclerosis Patients Treated with the Pregnancy Hormone Estriol," *The Journal of Immunology* 171, no. 11 (December 2003): 6267–6274.

98. Tomassini et al., "Sex Hormones Modulate Brain Damage."

99. Ibid.

100. S. M. Gold et al., "Immune Modulation and Increased Neurotrophic Factor Production in Multiple Sclerosis Patients Treated with Testosterone," *Journal of Neuroinflammation* 5, no. 32 (2008).

101. N. L. Sicotte et al., "Testosterone Treatment in Multiple Sclerosis: A Pilot Study," *Archives of Neurology* 64, no. 5 (May 2007): 683–688.

102. M. C. Ysrraelit et al., "Impaired Hypothalamic-Pituitary-Adrenal Axis Activity in Patients with Multiple Sclerosis," *Neurology* 71, no. 24 (December 2008): 1948–1954.

103. C. Heidbrink et al., "Reduced Cortisol Levels in Cerebrospinal Fluid and Differential Distribution of 11β-Hydroxysteroid Dehydrogenases in Multiple Sclerosis: Implications for Lesion Pathogenesis," *Brain. Behavior, and Immunity* 24, no. 6 (August 2010): 975–984.

104. Tellez et al., "Fatigue in Progressive Multiple Sclerosis."

105. Suzuki et al., "Low Serum Levels of Dehydroepiandrosterone."

106. C. Du et al., "Administration of Dehydroepiandrosterone Suppresses Experimental Allergic Encephalomyelitis in SJL/J Mice," *Journal of Immunology* 167, no. 12 (December 2001): 7094–7101.

107. Voskuhl, *MS Connection Blog.*

108. "International Society for Neurofeedback and Research: Addictive Disorders Bibliography," *ISNR,* http://noviancounseling.wix.com/bibliography #!addictive-disorders/c1o0f.

109. Carrillo-Vico et al., "Melatonin: Buffering the Immune System."

110. McMurray and May, "Sex Hormones and Systemic Lupus Erythematosus."

111. Appenzeller et al., "Prevalence of Thyroid Dysfunction"; and Chan et al., "Thyroid Disease in Systemic Lupus Erythematosus."

112. Richardson, "Primer: Epigenetics of Autoimmunity."

113. Kapsimalis et al., "Cytokines and Normal Sleep"; and M. R. Opp, "Cytokines and Sleep," *Sleep Medicine Reviews* 9, no. 5 (October 2005): 355–364.

114. Majde and Krueger, "Links between the Innate Immune System."

115. A. Alberti et al., "Plasma Cytokine Levels in Patients with Obstructive Sleep Apnea Syndrome: A Preliminary Study," *Journal of Sleep Research* 12, no. 4 (December 2003): 305–311.

116. Opp, "Cytokines and Sleep."

117. Majde and Krueger, "Links between the Innate Immune System."

118. A. K. Artemiadis et al., "Stress as a Risk Factor for Multiple Sclerosis Onset or Relapse: A Systematic Review," *Neuroepidemiology* 36, no. 2 (2011): 109–120.

119. P. H. Black, "Central Nervous System-Immune System Interactions: Psychoneuroendocrinology of Stress and Its Immune Consequences," *Antimicrobial Agents and Chemotherapy* 38, no. 1 (January 1994): 1–6.

120. M. Maes et al., "The Effects of Psychological Stress on Humans: Increased Production of Pro-Inflammatory Cytokines and Th1-Like Response in Stress-Induced Anxiety," *Cytokine* 10, no. 4 (April 1998): 313–318.

121. Lutgendorff et al., "The Role of Microbiota and Probiotics."

122. M. M. Holmes and L. A. Galea, "Defensive Behavior and Hippocampal Cell Proliferation: Differential Modulation by Naltrexone during Stress," *Behavioral Neuroscience* 116, no. 1 (February 2002): 160–168; A. Ray et al., "Modulation by Naltrexone of Stress Induced Changes in Humoral Immune Responsiveness and Gastric Mucosal Integrity in Rats," *Physiology & Behavior* 51, no. 2 (February 1992): 293–296; Y. Shavit et al., "Opioid Peptides Mediate the Suppressive Effect of Stress on Natural Killer Cell Cytotoxicity," *Science* 223, no. 4632 (January 1984): 188–190; K. Briski et al., "Counteraction by Naltrexone of Stress-Induced TSH Release: Role of Noradrenergic System," *Proceedings of the Society for Experimental Biology and Medicine* 177, no. 2 (November 1984): 354–359; J. A. McCubbin et al., "Naltrexone Potentiates Glycemic Responses during Stress and Epinephrine Challenge in Genetically Obese Mice," *Psychosomatic Medicine* 51, no. 4 (July–August 1989): 441–448; and L. M. Cancela et al., "Chronic Stress Attenuation of Alpha 2-Adrenoreceptor Reactivity Is Reversed by Naltrexone," *Pharmacology Biochemistry and Behavior* 31, no. 1 (September 1988): 33–35.

123. G. I. Keshet and M. Weinstock, "Maternal Naltrexone Prevents Morphological and Behavioral Alterations Induced in Rats by Prenatal Stress," *Pharmacology Biochemistry and Behavior* 50, no. 3 (March 1995): 413–419.

124. L. D. Cowan et al., "Breast Cancer Incidence in Women with a History of Progesterone Deficiency," *American Journal of Epidemiology* 114, no. 2 (August 1981): 209–217.

125. Burns, "Ultra-Low-Dose Opioid Antagonists."

126. M. Gironi et al., "A Pilot Trial of Low-Dose Naltrexone in Primary Progressive Multiple Sclerosis," *Multiple Sclerosis* 14, no. 8 (September 2008): 1076–1083.

127. B. A. Cree et al., "Pilot Trial of Low-Dose Naltrexone and Quality of Life in Multiple Sclerosis," *Annals of Neurology* 68, no. 2 (August 2010): 145–150.

128. Lelu et al., "Estrogen Receptor α Signaling."

129. Ibid.

130. J. Starkey, "Want to Quit Smoking? Acupuncture Can Help You with Cravings," *Cleveland Clinic*, October 27, 2014, http://health.clevelandclinic.org/2014/10/want-to-quit-smoking-acupuncture-can-help-you-with-cravings/; and D. He et al., "Effect of Acupuncture on Smoking Cessation or Reduction: An 8-Month and 5-Year Follow-up Study," *Preventive Medicine* 33, no. 5 (November 2001): 364–372.

131. "International Society for Neurofeedback and Research: Addictive Disorders Bibliography"; and X. Li et al., "Volitional Reduction of Anterior Cingulate Cortex Activity Produces Decreased Cue Craving in Smoking Cessation: A Preliminary Real-Time fMRI Study," *Addiction Biology* 18, no. 4 (July 2013): 739–748.

132. Carrillo-Vico et al., "Melatonin: Buffering the Immune System."
133. G. J. Lin et al., "Modulation by Melatonin of the Pathogenesis of Inflammatory Autoimmune Diseases," *International Journal of Molecular Science* 14, no. 6 (June 2013): 11742–11766.

Chapter Three: Inflammatory Bowel Disease

1. D. Q. Shih and S. R. Targan, "Immunopathogenesis of Inflammatory Bowel Disease," *World Journal of Gastroenterology* 14, no. 3 (January 2008): 390–400.
2. J. M. Reimund et al., "Anti-Tumor Necrosis Factor-Alpha (TNF-alpha) Treatment Strategies in Crohn's Disease," *Recent Patents on Inflammation & Allergy Drug Discovery* 1, no. 1 (February 2007): 21–34.
3. S. R. Targan et al., "A Short-Term Study of Chimeric Monoclonal Antibody cA2 to Tumor Necrosis Factor Alpha for Crohn's Disease. Crohn's Disease cA2 Study Group," *New England Journal of Medicine* 337, no. 15 (October 1997): 1029–1035.
4. W. J. Sandborn and S. B. Hanauer, "Antitumor Necrosis Factor Therapy for Inflammatory Bowel Disease: A Review of Agents, Pharmacology, Clinical Results, and Safety," *Inflammatory Bowel Diseases* 5, no. 2 (May 1999): 119–133.
5. M. Toruner et al., "Risk Factors for Opportunistic Infections in Patients with Inflammatory Bowel Disease," *Gastroenterology* 134, no. 4 (April 2008): 929–936; and R. Panaccione et al., "Review Article: Treatment Algorithms to Maximize Remission and Minimize Corticosteroid Dependence in Patients with Inflammatory Bowel Disease," *Alimentary Pharmacology & Therapeutics* 28, no. 6 (September 2008): 674–688.
6. A. C. Mackey et al., "Hepatosplenic T Cell Lymphoma Associated with Infliximab Use in Young Patients Treated for Inflammatory Bowel Disease," *Journal of Pediatric Gastroenterology and Nutrition* 44, no. 2 (February 2007): 265–267.
7. L. J. Ghazi et al., "Step Up Versus Early Biologic Therapy for Crohn's Disease in Clinical Practice," *Inflammatory Bowel Disorders* 19, no. 7 (June 2013): 1397–1403; and W. Reinisch et al., "Recommendations for the Treatment of Ulcerative Colitis with Infliximab: A Gastroenterology Expert Group Consensus," *Journal of Crohn's and Colitis* 6, no. 2 (March 2012): 248–258.
8. H. Sokol et al., "Usefulness of Co-Treatment with Immunomodulators in Patients with Inflammatory Bowel Disease Treated with Scheduled Infliximab Maintenance Therapy," *Gut* 59, no. 10 (October 2010): 1363–1368; T. Dassopoulos and C. A. Sninsky, "Optimizing Immunomodulators and Anti-TNF Agents in the Therapy of Crohn Disease," *Gastroenterology Clinics of North America* 41, no. 2 (June 2012): 393–409; and J. F. Colombel et al., "Infliximab, Azathioprine, or Combination Therapy for Crohn's Disease," *New England Journal of Medicine* 362, no. 15 (April 2010): 1383–1395.
9. G. R. Lichtenstein et al., "Serious Infection and Mortality in Patients with Crohn's Disease: More Than 5 Years of Follow-up in the TREAT™ Registry," *American Journal of Gastroenterology* 107, no. 9 (September 2012): 1409–1422.

10. D. Phillippe et al., "Mu Opioid Receptor Expression Is Increased in Inflammatory Bowel Diseases: Implications for Homeostatic Intestinal Inflammation," *Gut* 55, no. 6 (June 2006): 815–823.

11. M. Waldhoer et al., "Opioid Receptors," *Annual Review of Biochemistry* 73 (2004): 953–990.

12. P. S. Portoghese et al., "Identity of the Putative Delta1-Opioid Receptor as a Delta-Kappa Heteromer in the Mouse Spinal Cord," *European Journal of Pharmacology* 467, nos. 1–3 (April 2003): 233–234; B. M. Sharp, "Multiple Opioid Receptors on Immune Cells Modulate Intracellular Signalling," *Brain, Behavior, and Immunity* 20, no. 1 (January 2006): 9–14; and S. Suzuki et al., "Interactions of Opioid and Chemokine Receptors: Oligomerization of Mu, Kappa, And Delta with CCR5 on Immune Cells," *Experimental Cell Research* 280, no. 2 (November 2002): 192–200.

13. G. Parenty et al., "CXCR2 Chemokine Receptor Antagonism Enhances DOP Opioid Receptor Function via Allosteric Regulation of the CXCR2-DOP Receptor Heterodimer," *Biochemical Journal* 412, no. 2 (June 2008): 245–256; and F. A. White et al., "Chemokines: Integrators of Pain and Inflammation," *Nature Reviews Drug Discovery* 4, no. 10 (October 2005): 834–844.

14. T. J. Rogers and P. K. Peterson, "Opioid G Protein-Coupled Receptors: Signals at the Crossroads of Inflammation," *Trends in Immunology* 24, no. 3 (2003): 116–121; and O. M. Pello et al., "Ligand Stabilization of CXCR4/Delta-Opioid Receptor Heterodimers Reveals a Mechanism for Immune Response Regulation," *European Journal of Immunology* 38, no. 2 (February 2008): 537–549.

15. Geraldine Parenty, Shirley Appelbe, and Graeme Milligan, "CXR2 Chemokine Receptor Antagonism enhances DOP Opioid Receptor Function," *Biochemical Journal* (June 2008). doi: 10.1042/BJ20071689

16. N. Zhang and J. J. Oppenheim, "Crosstalk between Chemokines and Neuronal Receptors Bridges Immune and Nervous Systems," *Journal of Leukocyte Biology* 78, no. 6 (December 2005): 1210–1214.

17. Parenty et al., "CXCR2 Chemokine Receptor Antagonism."

18. Phillippe et al., "Mu Opioid Receptor Expression."

19. I. S. Zagon et al., "Immunoelectron Microscopic Localization of the Opioid Growth Factor Receptor (OGFr) and OGF in the Cornea," *Brain Research* 967 (2003): 37–47.

20. Ibid.

21. N. A. Shahabi et al., "Expression of Delta Opioid Receptors by Splenocytes from SEB-Treated Mice and Effects on Phosphorylation of MAP Kinase," *Cellular Immunology* 205, no. 2 (November 2000): 84–93.

22. Q. Wang et al., "Methionine Enkephalin (MENK) Improves Lymphocyte Subpopulations in Human Peripheral Blood of 50 Cancer Patients by Inhibiting Regulatory T Cells (Tregs)," *Human Vaccines & Immunotherapeutics* 10, no. 7 (2014): 1836–1840.

23. K. J. Gross and C. Pothoulakis, "Role of Neuropeptides in Inflammatory Bowel Disease," *Inflammatory Bowel Diseases* 13, no. 7 (2007): 918–932; and P. Holzer,

"Opioid Receptors in the Gastrointestinal Tract," *Regulatory Peptides* 155, nos. 1–3 (June 2009): 11–17.

24. I. S. Zagon and P. J. Mclaughlin, "Targeting Opioid Signaling in Crohn's Disease: New Therapeutic Pathways," *Expert Review of Gastroenterology & Hepatology* 5, no. 5 (October 2011): 555–558.

25. Ibid.

26. I. S. Zagon et al., "B Lymphocyte Proliferation Is Suppressed by the opioid Growth Factor-Opioid Growth Factor Receptor Axis: Implication for the Treatment of Autoimmune Diseases," *Immunobiology* 216, nos. 1–2 (January–February 2011): 173–183; and I. S. Zagon et al., "T Lymphocyte Proliferation Is Suppressed by the Opioid Growth Factor ([Met(5)]-Enkephalin)-Opioid Growth Factor Receptor Axis: Implication for the Treatment of Autoimmune Diseases," *Immunobiology* 216, no. 5 (May 2011): 579–590.

27. G. L. Matters et al., "The Opioid Antagonist Naltrexone Improves Murine Inflammatory Bowel Disease," *Journal of Immunotoxicology* 5, no. 2 (April 2008): 179–187.

28. J. Ninković and S. Roy, "Role of the Mu-Opioid Receptor in Opioid Modulation of Immune Function," *Amino Acids* 45, no. 1 (July 2013): 9–24.

29. K. S. Iwaszkiewicz et al., "Targeting Peripheral Opioid Receptors to Promote Analgesic and Anti-inflammatory Actions," *Frontiers in Pharmacology* 4 (October 2013): 132.

30. J. Meng et al., "Morphine Induces Bacterial Translocation in Mice by Compromising Intestinal Barrier Function in a TLR-Dependent Manner," *PLOS One* 8, no. 1 (2013).

31. A. E. Østvik et al., "Expression of Toll-Like Receptor-3 Is Enhanced in Active Inflammatory Bowel Disease and Mediates the Excessive Release of Lipocalin 2," *Clinical & Experimental Immunology* 173, no. 3 (September 2013): 502–511.

32. J. Younger, L. Parkitny, and D. McLain, "The Use of Low-Dose Naltrexone (LDN) as a Novel Anti-inflammatory Treatment for Chronic Pain," *Clinical Rheumatology* 33 (2014): 451–459.

33. J. M. Davies and M. T. Abreu, "Host-Microbe Interactions in the Small Bowel," *Current Opinion in Gastroenterology* 31, no. 2 (March 2015): 118–123.

34. J. P. Smith et al., "Low-Dose Naltrexone Therapy Improves Active Crohn's Disease," *American Journal of Gastroenterology* 102, no. 4 (April 2007): 820–828.

35. J. P. Smith et al., "Therapy with the Opioid Antagonist Naltrexone Promotes Mucosal Healing in Active Crohn's Disease: A Randomized Placebo-Controlled Trial," *Digestive Diseases and Sciences* 56, no. 7 (July 2011): 2088–2097.

36. A. Shannon et al., "Low-Dose Naltrexone for Treatment of Duodenal Crohn's Disease in a Pediatric Patient," *Inflammatory Bowel Diseases* 16, no. 9 (September 2010): 1457; and J. P. Smith et al., "Safety and Tolerability of Low-Dose Naltrexone Therapy in Children with Moderate to Severe Crohn's Disease: A Pilot Study," *Journal of Clinical Gastroenterology* 47, no. 4 (April 2013): 339–345.

37. Smith et al., "Therapy with the Opioid Antagonist Naltrexone."

38. Ibid.

39. S. Nathoo and S. C. Glover, "Low-Dose Naltrexone in the Treatment of Crohn's Disease: A Case Series," *Gastroenterology* 184, no. 4 (April 2015).

40. L. B. Weinstock, "Naltrexone Therapy for Crohn's Disease and Ulcerative Colitis," *Journal of Clinical Gastroenterology* 48, no. 8 (September 2014): 742.

41. Ibid.

42. Smith et al., "Therapy with the Opioid Antagonist Naltrexone."

43. Ibid.

44. Ibid.

45. J. Ploesser et al., "Low Dose Naltrexone: Side Effects and Efficacy in Gastrointestinal Disorders," *International Journal of Pharmaceutical Compounding* 14, no. 2 (March/April 2010): 171–173.

46. Matters et al., "The Opioid Antagonist Naltrexone Improves."

47. R. N. Donahue et al., "Low-Dose Naltrexone Targets the Opioid Growth Factor-Opioid Growth Factor Receptor Pathway to Inhibit Cell Proliferation: Mechanistic Evidence from a Tissue Culture Model," *Experimental Biology and Medicine (Maywood)* 236, no. 9 (September 2011): 1036–1050.

48. S. Garud et al., "Meta-Analysis of the Placebo Response in Ulcerative Colitis," *Digestive Diseases and Sciences* 53, no. 4 (April 2008): 875–891.

Chapter Four: Chronic Fatigue Syndrome and Fibromyalgia

1. G. E. Ehrlich, "Pain Is Real; Fibromyalgia Isn't," *The Journal of Rheumatology* 30, no. 8 (August 2003): 1666–1667; F. Wolfe, "Stop Using the American College of Rheumatology Criteria in the Clinic," *The Journal of Rheumatology* 30, no. 8 (August 2003): 1671–1672; and H. A. Smythe, "Fibromyalgia Among Friends," *The Journal of Rheumatology* 31, no. 4 (April 2004): 627–630.

2. Ehrlich, "Pain Is Real"; Wolfe, "Stop Using the American College of Rheumatology"; and Smythe, "Fibromyalgia Among Friends."

3. K. Holtorf, "Diagnosis and Treatment of Hypothalamic-Pituitary-Adrenal (HPA) Axis Dysfunction in Patients with Chronic Fatigue Syndrome (CFS) and Fibromyalgia (FM)," *Journal of Chronic Fatigue Syndrome* 14, no. 3 (2008); W. Riedel et al., "Secretory Pattern of GH, TSH, Thyroid Hormones, ACTH, Cortisol, FSH, and LH in Patients with Fibromyalgia Syndrome Following Systemic Injection of the Relevant Hypothalamic-Releasing Hormones," *Zeitschrift für Rheumatologie* 57 (1998): 81–87; G. Neeck and W. Riedel, "Thyroid Functions in Patients with Fibromyalgia Syndrome," *The Journal of Rheumatology* 19, no. 7 (1992): 1120–1122; and G. Neeck and W. Riedel, "Neuromediator and Hormonal Perturbations in Fibromyalgia Syndrome: Results of Chronic Stress?," *Baillière's Clinical Rheumatology* 8, no. 4 (1994): 763–775.

4. Anthony L. Komaroff et al., "Health Status in Patients with Chronic Fatigue Syndrome," The American Journal of Medicine, (September, 1996). doi: 10.1016/S0002.

5. Committee on the Diagnostic Criteria for Myalgic Encephalomyelitis/ Chronic Fatigue Syndrome, "Beyond Myalgic Encephalomyelitis/Chronic

Fatigue Syndrome: Redefining an Illness," *Institute of Medicine of the National Academies* 2015.

6. M. M. Andersen et al., "Illness and Disability in Danish Chronic Fatigue Syndrome Patients at Diagnosis and 5-Year Follow-up," *Journal of Psychosomatic Research* 56, no. 2 (February 2004): 217–229.

7. C. H. Bombardier and D. Buchwald, "Outcome and Prognosis of Patients with Chronic Fatigue vs Chronic Fatigue Syndrome," *Archives of Internal Medicine* 155, no. 19 (October 1995): 2105–2110.

8. F. Wolfe et al, "Health Status and Disease Severity in Fibromyalgia: Results of a Six-Center Longitudinal Study," *Arthritis & Rheumatology* 40, no. 9 (September 1997): 1571–1579.

9. J. Joyce et al., "The Prognosis of Chronic Fatigue and Chronic Fatigue Syndrome: A Systematic Review," *QJM: An International Journal of Medicine* 90, no. 3 (March 1997): 223–233.

10. J. Bowen et al., "Chronic Fatigue Syndrome: A Survey of GPs' Attitudes and Knowledge," *Family Practice* 22, no. 4 (August 2005): 389–393.

11. M. A. Thomas and A. P. Smith, "Primary Healthcare Provision and Chronic Fatigue Syndrome: A Survey of Patients' and General Practitioners' Beliefs," *BMC Family Practice* 13 (December 2005).

12. Bombardier and Buchwald, "Outcome and Prognosis of Patients."

13. J. E. Teitelbaum et al., "Effective Treatment of Chronic Fatigue Syndrome and Fibromyalgia—A Randomized, Double-Blind, Placebo-Controlled, Intent-to-Treat Study," *Journal of Chronic Fatigue Syndrome* 8, no. 2 (2000).

14. Holtorf, "Diagnosis and Treatment of Hypothalamic-Pituitary-Adrenal (HPA)."

15. Ibid.

16. Ibid.

17. Ibid.

18. K. Holtorf, "A Confounding Condition: Treating Chronic Fatigue Syndrome and Fibromyalgia Requires Addressing the Underlying Problems," *Healthy Aging* 4, no. 4 (November/December 2008): 1–8.

19. Teitelbaum et al., "Effective Treatment of Chronic Fatigue Syndrome"; and Holtorf, "Diagnosis and Treatment of Hypothalamic-Pituitary-Adrenal (HPA)."

20. J. Younger and S. Mackey, "Fibromyalgia Symptoms Are Reduced by Low-Dose Naltrexone: A Pilot Study," *Pain Medicine* 10, no. 4 (May–June 2009): 663–672.

21. J. Younger et al., "Low-Dose Naltrexone for the Treatment of Fibromyalgia: Findings of a Small, Randomized, Double-Blind, Placebo-Controlled, Counterbalanced, Crossover Trial Assessing Daily Pain Levels," *Arthritis & Rheumatology* 65, no. 2 (February 2013): 529–538.

Chapter Five: Thyroid Disorders

1. A.C. Bianco et al., "Biochemistry, Cellular and Molecular Biology, and Physiological Roles of the Iodothyronine Selenodeiodinases," *Endocrine Reviews* 23, no. 1 (February 2002): 38–89; J. E. Silva and P. R. Larsen, "Pituitary

Nuclear 3,5,3'-Triiodothyronine and Thyrotropin Secretion: An Explanation for the Effect of Thyroxine," *Science* 198, no. 4317 (November 1997): 617–620; R. J. Koenig et al., "Regulation of Thyroxine 5'-Deiodinase Activity by 3,5,3'-Triiodothyronine in Cultured Rat Anterior Pituitary Cells," *Endocrinology* 115, no. 1 (July 1984): 324–329; J. E. Silva et al., "The Contribution of Local Tissue Thyroxine Monodeiodination to the Nuclear 3,5,3'-Triiodothyronine in Pituitary, Liver, and Kidney of Euthyroid Rats," *Endocrinology* 103, no. 4 (October 1978): 1196–1207; T. J. Visser et al., "Evidence for Two Pathways of Iodothyronine 5'-Deiodination in Rat Pituitary That Differ in Kinetics, Propylthiouracil Sensitivity, and Response to Hypothyroidism," *The Journal of Clinical Investigation* 71, no. 4 (April 1983): 992–1002; P. R. Larsen et al., "Relationships between Circulating and Intracellular Thyroid Hormones: Physiological and Clinical Implications," *Endocrine Reviews* 2, no. 1 (Winter 1981): 87–102; M. M. Kaplan, "The Role of Thyroid Hormone Deiodination in the Regulation of Hypothalamo-Pituitary Function," *Neuroendocrinology* 38, no. 3 (March 1984): 254–260; R. P. Peeters et al., "Tissue Thyroid Hormone Levels in Critical Illness," *The Journal of Clinical Endocrinology & Metabolism* 90, no. 12 (December 2005): 6498–6507; and R. P. Peeters et al., "Serum 3,3',5'-Triiodothyronine (rT3) and 3,5,3'-Triiodothyronine/Rt3 Are Prognostic Markers in Critically Ill Patients and Are Associated with Postmortem Tissue Deiodinase Activities," *The Journal of Clinical Endocrinology & Metabolism* 90, no. 8 (August 2005): 4559–4565.

2. Bianco et al., "Biochemistry, Cellular and Molecular Biology."

3. I. J. Chopra et al., "Reciprocal Changes in Serum Concentrations of 3,3',5-Triiodothyronine (T3) in Systemic Illnesses," *The Journal of Clinical Endocrinology & Metabolism* 41, no. 6 (December 1975): 1043–1049.

4. M. Linnoila et al., "High Reverse T3 Levels in Manic and Unipolar Depressed Women," *Psychiatry Research* 6, no. 3 (June 1982): 271–276.

5. R. L. Araujo et al., "Tissue-Specific Deiodinase Regulation during Food Restriction and Low Replacement Dose of Leptin in Rats," *American Journal of Physiology—Endocrinology and Metabolism* 295, no. 5 (May 2009): 1157–1563.

6. M. Krotkiewski et al., "Small Doses of Triiodothyronine Can Change Some Risk Factors Associated with Abdominal Obesity," *International Journal of Obesity and Related Metabolic Disorders* 21, no. 10 (October 1997): 922–929.

7. S. Islam et al., "A Comparative Study of Thyroid Hormone Levels in Diabetic and Non-diabetic Patients," *The Southeast Asian Journal of Tropical Medicine and Public Health* 39, no. 5 (September 2008): 913–916.

8. R. Docter et al., "The Sick Euthyroid Syndrome: Changes in Thyroid Hormone Serum Parameters and Hormone Metabolism," *Clinical Endocrinology (Oxford)* 39, no. 5 (Nov. 1993): 499–518.

9. J. C. Lowe et al., "Effectiveness and Safety of T3 (Triiodothyronine) Therapy for Euthyroid Fibromyalgia: A Double-Blind Placebo-Controlled Response-Driven Crossover Study," *Clinical Bulletin of Myofascial Therapy* 2, nos. 2–3 (1997): 31–58.

10. L. Krulich et al., "On the Role of the Central Noradrenergic and Dopaminergic Systems in the Regulation of TSH Secretion in the Rat," *Endocrinology* 100, no. 2 (February 1977): 496–505.

11. K. Moriyama et al., "Thyroid Hormone Action Is Disrupted by Bisphenol A as an Antagonist," *The Journal of Clinical Endocrinology & Metabolism* 87, no. 11 (November 2002): 5185–5190.

12. L. J. De Groot, "Non-thyroidal Illness Syndrome Is a Manifestation of Hypothalamic-Pituitary Dysfunction, and in View of Current Evidence, Should Be Treated with Appropriate Replacement Therapies," *Critical Care Clinics* 22, no. 1 (January 2006): 57–86.

13. K. Miyashita et al., "Regulation of Rat Liver Type 1 Iodothyronine Deiodinase mRNA Levels by Testosterone," *Molecular and Cellular Endocrinology* 115, no. 2 (December 1995): 161–167.

14. J. U. Schilling et al., "Low T3 Syndrome in Multiple Trauma Patients—A Phenomenon or Important Pathogenetic Factor?," *Medizinische Klinik (Munich)* 94 (October 1999): 66–69.

15. Bianco et al., "Biochemistry, Cellular and Molecular Biology."

16. Ibid.

17. J. E. Silva et al., "Qualitative and Quantitative Differences in the Pathways of Extrathyroidal Triiodothyronine Generation between Euthyroid and Hypothyroid Rats," *The Journal of Clinical Investigation* 73, no. 4 (April 1984): 898–907.

18. D. Salvatore et al., "Molecular Biological and Biochemical Characterization of the Human Type 2 Selenodeiodinase," *Endocrinology* 137, no. 8 (August 1996): 3308–3315.

19. Silva et al., "The Contribution of Local Tissue Thyroxine Monodeiodination."

20. M. Schimmel and R. D. Utiger, "Thyroidal and Peripheral Production of Thyroid Hormones: Review of Recent Findings and Their Clinical Implications," *Annals of Internal Medicine* 87, no. 6 (December 1977): 760–768.

21. Kaplan, "The Role of Thyroid Hormone Deiodination."

22. Silva et al., "The Contribution of Local Tissue Thyroxine Monodeiodination."

23. Koenig et al., "Regulation of Thyroxine 5'-Deiodinase Activity."

24. A. R. Harris et al., "Effect of Starvation, Nutriment Replacement, and Hypothyroidism on in Vitro Hepatic T4 to T3 Conversion in the Rat," *Metabolism* 27, no. 11 (November 1978): 1680–1690.

25. Peeters et al., 2005.

26. Chopra et al., "Reciprocal Changes in Serum Concentrations."

27. V. S. Lim et al., "Reduced Triiodothyronine Content in Liver But Not Pituitary of the Uremic Rat Model: Demonstration of Changes Compatible with Thyroid Hormone Deficiency in Liver Only," *Endocrinology* 114, no.1 (January 1984): 280–286.

28. Ibid.

29. P. R. Larsen, "Thyroid-Pituitary Interaction: Feedback Regulation of Thyrotropin Secretion by Thyroid Hormones," *New England Journal of Medicine* 306, no. 1 (January 1982): 23–32.

30. Ibid.
31. Kaplan, "The Role of Thyroid Hormone Deiodination."
32. Peeters et al., "Serum 3,3',5'-Triiodothyronine (rT3)."
33. R. Okamoto and D. Leibfritz, "Adverse Effects of Reverse Triiodothyronine on Cellular Metabolism as Assessed by 1H and 31P NMR Spectroscopy," *Research in Experimental Medicine* 197, no. 4 (1997): 211–217.
34. A. Sechman et al., "The Relationship between Basal Metabolic Rate (BMR) and Concentrations of Plasma Thyroid Hormones in Fasting Cockerels," *Folia Biologica (Krawkow)* 31, nos. 1–2 (1989): 83–90.
35. Silva et al., "The Contribution of Local Tissue Thyroxine Monodeiodination."
36. A. M. Mitchell et al., "Uptake of Reverse T3 in the Human Choriocarcinoma Cell Line, JAr," *Placenta* 20, no. 1 (January 1999): 65–70.
37. Kaplan, "The Role of Thyroid Hormone Deiodination."
38. Bianco et al., "Biochemistry, Cellular and Molecular Biology."
39. Ibid.; and Peeters et al., "Serum 3,3',5'-Triiodothyronine (rT3)."
40. Ibid.
41. Okamoto and Leibfritz, "Adverse Effects of Reverse Triiodothyronine."
42. G. A. Brent and J. M. Hershman, "Thyroxine Therapy in Patients with Severe Nonthyroidal Illnesses and Low Serum Thyroxine Concentration," *The Journal of Clinical Endocrinology & Metabolism* 63, no. 1 (July 1986): 1–8.
43. Krotkiewski et al., "Small Doses of Triiodothyronine Can Change."
44. M. E. Everts et al., "Different Regulation of Thyroid Hormone Transport in Liver and Pituitary: Its Possible Role in the Maintenance of Low T3 Production during Nonthyroidal Illness and Fasting in Man," *Thyroid* 6, no. 4 (August 1996): 359–368; M. E. Everts et al., "Uptake of Thyroxine in Cultured Anterior Pituitary Cells of Euthyroid Rats," *Endocrinology* 134, no. 6 (1994): 2490–2497; G. Hennemann and E. P. Krenning, "The Kinetics of Thyroid Hormone Transporters and Their Role in Non-thyroidal Illness and Starvation," *Best Practice & Research Clinical Endocrinology* 21, no. 2 (June 2007): 323–328; F. W. Wassen et al., "Thyroid Hormone Uptake in Cultured Rat Anterior Pituitary Cells: Effects of Energy Status and Bilirubin," *Journal of Endocrinology* 165, no. 3 (June 2000): 599–606; E. Krenning et al., "Characteristics of Active Transport of Thyroid Hormone into Rat Hepatocytes," *Biochimica et Biophysica Acta* 676, no. 3 (September 1981): 314–320; D. L. St. Germain and V. A. Galton, "Comparative Study of Pituitary-Thyroid Hormone Economy in Fasting and Hypothyroid Rats," *The Journal of Clinical Investigation* 75, no. 2 (February 1985): 679–688; Lim et al., "Reduced Triiodothyronine Content in Liver"; M. E. Everts et al., "Effects of a Furan Fatty Acid and Indoxyl Sulfate on Thyroid Hormone Uptake in Cultured Anterior Pituitary Cells," *American Journal of Physiology* 268, no. 5 pt. 1 (May 1995): 974–979; and L. Kragie and D. Doyle, "Benzodiazepines Inhibit Temperature-Dependent L-[125I]triiodothyronine Accumulation into Human Liver, Human Neuroblast, and Rat Pituitary Cell Lines," *Endocrinology* 130, no. 3 (March 1992): 1211–1216.
45. M. E. Everts et al., "Different Regulation of Thyroid Hormone Transport in Liver and Pituitary: Its Possible Role in the Maintenance of Low T3 Production

during Nonthyroidal Illness and Fasting in Man," *Thyroid* 6, no. 4 (August 1996): 359–368; Hennemann and Krenning, "The Kinetics of Thyroid Hormone Transporters"; St. Germain and Galton, "Comparative Study of Pituitary-Thyroid Hormone Economy"; Kragie and Doyle, "Benzodiazepines Inhibit Temperature-Dependent"; and R. Arem et al., "Reduced Tissue Thyroid Hormone Levels in Fatal Illness," *Metabolism* 42, no. 9 (September 1993): 1102–1108.

46. Everts et al., "Different Regulation of Thyroid Hormone Transport."

47. Chopra et al., "Reciprocal Changes in Serum Concentrations."

48. Bianco et al., "Biochemistry, Cellular and Molecular Biology"; Peeters et al., "Serum 3,3',5'-Triiodothyronine (rT3)"; and R. P. Peeters et al., "Reduced Activation and Increased Inactivation of Thyroid Hormone in Tissues of Critically Ill Patients," *The Journal of Clinical Endocrinology & Metabolism* 88, no. 7 (July 2003): 3202–3211.

49. Ibid.

50. Chopra et al., "Reciprocal Changes in Serum Concentrations."

51. G. Brabant et al., "Circadian and Pulsatile Thyrotropin Secretion in Euthyroid Man under the Influence of Thyroid Hormone and Glucocorticoid Administration," *The Journal of Clinical Endocrinology & Metabolism* 65, no. 1 (July 1987): 83–88.

52. I. M. Jackson, "The Thyroid Axis and Depression," *Thyroid* 8, no. 10 (October 1998): 951–956.

53. R. G. Cooke et al., "T3 Augmentation of Antidepressant Treatment in T4-Replaced Thyroid Patients," *Journal of Clinical Psychiatry* 53, no. 1 (January 1992): 16–18.

54. M. H. Samuels et al., "Health Status, Psychological Symptoms, Mood, and Cognition in L-Thyroxine-Treated Hypothyroid Subjects," *Thyroid* 17, no. 3 (March 2007): 249–258.

55. D. H. Sarne and S. Refetoff, "Measurement of Thyroxine Uptake from Serum by Cultured Human Hepatocytes as an Index of Thyroid Status: Reduced Thyroxine Uptake from Serum of Patients with Nonthyroidal Illness," *The Journal of Clinical Endocrinology & Metabolism* 61, no. 6 (December 1985): 1046–1052.

56. Ibid.

57. Everts et al., "Effects of a Furan Fatty Acid"; and C. F. Lim et al., "Inhibition of Thyroxine Transport into Cultured Rat Hepatocytes by Serum of Non-uremic Critically Ill Patients: Effects of Bilirubin and Nonesterified Fatty Acids," *The Journal of Clinical Endocrinology & Metabolism* 76, no. 5 (May 1993): 1165–1172.

58. Wassen et al., "Thyroid Hormone Uptake."

59. Arem et al., "Reduced Tissue Thyroid Hormone Levels."

60. G. A. Cremaschi et al., "Chronic Stress Influences the Immune System through the Thyroid Axis," *Life Sciences* 67, no. 26 (November 2000): 3171–3179.

61. I. J. Chopra et al., "Opposite Effects of Dexamethasone on Serum Concentrations of 3,3',5'-Triiodothyronine (Reverse T3) and 3,3',5-Triiodothyronine (T3)," *The Journal of Clinical Endocrinology & Metabolism* 41, no. 5 (November 1975): 911–920.

62. F. Undén et al., "Twenty-Four-Hour Serum Levels of T4 and T3 in Relation to Decreased TSH Serum Levels and Decreased TSH Response to TRH in Affective Disorders," *Acta Psychiatrica Scandinavica* 73, no. 4 (April 1986): 358–365.

63. Linnoila et al., "High Reverse T3 Levels."

64. Okamoto and Leibfritz, "Adverse Effects of Reverse Triiodothyronine."

65. Mitchell et al., "Uptake of Reverse T3."

66. G. M. Sullivan et al., "Low Levels of Transthyretin in CSF of Depressed Patients," *The American Journal of Psychiatry* 156, no. 5 (May 1999): 710–715; and J. A. Hatterer et al., "CSF Transthyretin in Patients with Depression," *The American Journal of Psychiatry* 150, no. 5 (May 1993): 813–815.

67. M. Linnoila et al., "Thyroid Hormones and TSH, Prolactin and LH Responses to Repeated TRH and LRH Injections in Depressed Patients," *Acta Psychiatrica Scandinavica* 59, no. 5 (May 1979): 536–544.

68. Jackson, "The Thyroid Axis and Depression"; C. Kirkegaard and J. Faber, "Altered Serum Levels of Thyroxine, Triiodothyronines and Diiodothyronines in Endogenous Depression," *Acta Endocrinologica (Copenhagen)* 96, no. 2 (February 1981): 199–207; Sullivan et al., "Low Levels of Transthyretin in CSF"; and Hatterer et al., "CSF Transthyretin in Patients."

69. Brabant et al., "Circadian and Pulsatile Thyrotropin Secretion"; P. C. Whybrow et al., "Thyroid Function and the Response to Liothyronine in Depression," *Archives of General Psychiatry* 26, no. 3 (March 1972): 242–245; Cooke et al., "T3 Augmentation of Antidepressant Treatment"; R. T. Joffe, "A Perspective on the Thyroid and Depression," *Canadian Journal of Psychiatry* 35, no. 9 (December 1990): 745–758; A. M. Sawka et al., "Does a Combination Regimen of Thyroxine (T4) and 3,5,3'-Triiodothyronine Improved Depressive Symptoms Better Than T4 Alone in Patients with Hypothyroidism? Results of a Double-Blind, Randomized, Controlled Trial," *The Journal of Clinical Endocrinology & Metabolism* 88, no. 10 (October 2003): 4551–4555; R. Cooper-Kazaz et al., "Combined Treatment with Sertraline and Liothyronine in Major Depression," *Archives of General Psychiatry* 64, no. 6 (June 2007): 679–688; and T. Kelly and D. Z. Lieberman, "The Use of Triiodothyronine as an Augmentation Agent in Treatment Resistant Bipolar II and Bipolar Disorder NOS," *Journal of Affective Disorders* 116, no. 3 (August 2009): 222–226.

70. M. Posternak et al., "A Pilot Effectiveness Study: Placebo-Controlled Trial of Adjunctive L-Triiodothyronine (T3) Used to Accelerate and Potentiate the Antidepressant Response," *International Journal of Neuropsychopharmacology* 11, no. 1 (February 2008): 15–25.

71. Kelly and Lieberman, "The Use of Triiodothyronine."

72. A. A. Nierenberg et al., "A Comparison of Lithium and T3 Augmentation Following Two Failed Medication Treatments for Depression: A STAR*D Report," *The American Journal of Psychiatry* 163, no. 9 (September 2006): 1519–1530.

73. Ibid.

74. J. E. Morley, "The Endocrinology of the Opiates and Opioid Peptides," *Metabolism* 30, no. 2 (February 1981): 195–209.

75. Krulich et al., "On the Role of the Central Noradrenergic."

76. Morley, "The Endocrinology of the Opiates."

77. Ibid.

78. A. B. Loucks and E. M. Heath, "Induction of Low-T3 Syndrome in Exercising Women Occurs at the Threshold of Energy Availability," *The American Journal of Physiology* 266, no. 3 pt. 2 (March 1994): 817–823.

79. K. D. Brownell et al., "The Effects of Repeated Cycles of Weight Loss and Regain in Rats," *Physiology & Behavior* 38, no. 4 (October 1986): 459–464.

80. C. F. Lim et al., "Transport of Thyroxine into Cultured Hepatocytes: Effects of Mild Nonthyroidal Illness and Calorie Restriction in Obese Subjects," *Clinical Endocrinology (Oxford)* 40, no. 1 (January 1994): 79–85.

81. J. T. van der Heyden et al., "Effects of Caloric Deprivation on Thyroid Hormone Tissue Uptake and Generation of Low-T3 Syndrome," *The American Journal of Physiology* 251, no. 2 pt. 1 (August 1986): 156–163.

82. R. L. Leibel and J. Hirsch, "Diminished Energy Requirements in Reduced-Obese Patients," *Metabolism* 33, no. 2 (February 1984): 164–170; M. S. Croxson and H. K. Ibbertson, "Low Serum Triiodothyronine (T3) and Hypothyroidism," *The Journal of Clinical Endocrinology & Metabolism* 44, no. 1 (January 1977): 167–174; Lim et al ., "Inhibition of Thyroxine Transport"; D. L. Elliot et al., "Sustained Depression of the Resting Metabolic Rate after Massive Weight Loss," *The American Journal of Clinical Nutrition* 49, no. 1 (January 1989): 93–96; M. M. Manore et al., "Energy Expenditure at Rest and during Exercise in Nonobese Female Cyclical Dieters and in Nondieting Control Subjects," *The American Journal of Clinical Nutrition* 54, no. 1 (July 1991): 41–46; C. F. Lim et al., "A Furan Fatty Acid and Indoxyl Sulfate Are the Putative Inhibitors of Thyroxine Hepatocyte Transport in Uremia," *The Journal of Clinical Endocrinology & Metabolism* 76, no. 2 (February 1993): 318–324; A. Brehm et al., "Increased Lipid Availability Impairs Insulin-Stimulated ATP Synthesis in Human Skeletal Muscle," *Diabetes* 55, no. 1 (January 2006): 136–140; N. M. DiMarco et al., "Effect of Fasting on Free Fatty Acid, Glycerol and Cholesterol Concentrations in Blood Plasma and Lipoprotein Lipase Activity in Adipose Tissue of Cattle," *Journal of Animal Science* 52, no. 1 (January 1981): 75–82; and S. N. Steen et al., "Metabolic Effects of Repeated Weight and Regain in Adolescent Wrestlers," *JAMA* 260, no. 1 (July 1988): 47–50.

83. E. Dillman et al., "Hypothermia in Iron Deficiency Due to Altered Triiodithyroidine Metabolism," *The American Journal of Physiology* 239, no. 5 (November 1980): 377–381.

84. S. M. Smith et al., "In Vitro Hepatic Thyroid Hormone Deiodination in Iron-Deficient Rats: Effect of Dietary Fat," *Life Sciences* 53, no. 8 (1993): 603–609.

85. T. Nagaya et al., "A Potential Role of Activated NF-Kappa B in the Pathogenesis of Euthyroid Sick Syndrome," *The Journal of Clinical Investigation* 106, no. 3 (August 2000): 393–402.

86. D. Zhou et al., "Exposure to Physical and Psychological Stressors Elevates Plasma Interleukin-6: Relationship to the Activation of the

Hypothalamic–Pituitary–Adrenal Axis," *Endocrinology* 133, no. 6 (December 1993): 2523–2530.

87. J. S. Yudkin et al., "Inflammation, Obesity, Stress and Coronary Heart Disease: Is Interleukin-6 the Link?," *Atherosclerosis* 148, no. 2 (February 2000): 209–214.

88. S. Liu et al., "A Prospective Study of Inflammatory Cytokines and Diabetes Mellitus in a Multiethnic Cohort of Postmenopausal Women," *Archives of Internal Medicine* 167, no. 15 (August 2007): 1676–1685.

89. M. Maes, "Evidence for an Immune Response in Major Depression: A Review and Hypothesis," *Progress in Neuropsychopharmacology and Biological Psychiatry* 19, no. 1 (January 1995): 11–38.

90. J. Pfeilschifter et al., "Changes in Proinflamatory Cytokine Activity after Menopause," *Endocrine Reviews* 23, no. 1 (February 2002): 90–119.

91. R. W. Alexander, "Inflammation and Coronary Artery Disease," *The New England Journal of Medicine* 331, no. 7 (August 1994): 468–469.

92. G. T. Espersen et al., "Tumor Necrosis Factor-Alpha and Interleukin-2 in Plasma from Rheumatoid Arthritis Patients in Relation to Disease," *Clinical Rheumatology* 10, no. 4 (December 1991): 374–376.

93. M. C. Cohen and S. Cohen, "Cytokine Function: A Study in Biologic Diversity," *American Journal of Clinical Pathology* 105, no. 5 (May 1996): 589–598.

94. S. Takeshita et al., "Induction of IL-6 and IL-10 Production by Recombinant HIV-1 Envelope Glycoprotein 41 (gp41) in the THP-1 Human Monocytic Cell Line," *Cellular Immunology* 165, no. 2 (October 1995): 234–242.

95. B. N. Lee et al., "A Cytokine-Based Neuroimmunologic Mechanism of Cancer Related Symptoms," *Neuroimmunomodulation* 11, no. 5 (2004): 279–292.

96. F. J. de Jong et al., "The Association of Pohymorphism in the Type 1 and 2 Deiodinase Genes with Circulation Thyroid Hormone Parameters and Atrophy of the Medial Temporal Lobe," *The Journal of Clinical Endocrinology & Metabolism* 92, no. 2 (February 2007): 636–640.

97. Peeters et al., 2005.

98. K. Holtorf, "Peripheral Thyroid Hormone Conversion and Its Impact on TSH and Metabolic Activity," *Journal of Restorative Medicine* 3 (2014): 30–52.

99. K. Holtorf, "Thyroid Hormone Transport into Cellular Tissue," *Journal of Restorative Medicine* 3 (2014): 53–68.

Chapter Six: Restless Legs Syndrome

1. L. B. Weinstock et al., "Restless Legs Syndrome—Theoretical Roles of Inflammatory and Immune Mechanisms," *Sleep Medicine Review* 16, no. 4 (August 2012): 341–354.

2. R. P. Allen et al., "Restless Legs Syndrome Prevalence and Impact: REST General Population Study," *Archives of Internal Medicine* 165 (2005): 1286–1292.

3. L. Ferini-Strambi and S. Marelli, "Pharmacotherapy for Restless Legs Syndrome," *Expert Opinion on Pharmacotherapy* 15, no. 8 (June 2014): 1127–1138.

4. A. S. Walters and D. B. Rye, "Review of the Relationship of Restless Legs Syndrome and Periodic Limb Movements in Sleep to Hypertension, Heart Disease, and Stroke," *Sleep* 32, no. 5 (May 2009): 589–597.

5. J. R. Connor et al., "Neuropathological Examination Suggests Impaired Brain Iron Acquisition in Restless Legs Syndrome," *Neurology* 61, no. 3 (August 2003): 304–309; and S. Mizuno et al., "CSF Iron, Ferritin, and Transferrin Levels in Restless Legs Syndrome," *Journal of Sleep Research* 14, no. 1 (March 2005): 43–47.

6. C. Trenkwalder et al., "Recent Advances in the Diagnosis, Genetics, and Treatment of Restless Legs Syndrome," *Journal of Neurology* 256, no. 4 (April 2009): 539–553.

7. D. Garcia-Borreguero and A. M. Williams, "An Update on Restless Legs Syndrome (Willis-Ekbom Disease): Clinical Features, Pathogenesis and Treatment," *Current Opinion in Neurology* 27, no. 4 (August 2014): 493–501.

8. F. Gemignani et al., "Restless Legs Syndrome and Polyneuropathy," *Movement Disorders* 21, no. 8 (August 2006): 1254–1257; D. Lo Coco et al., "Restless Legs Syndrome in a Patient with Multifocal Motor Neuropathy," *Neurological Sciences* 30, no. 5 (October 2009): 401–403; and A. Nineb et al., "Restless Legs Syndrome Is Frequently Overlooked in Patients Being Evaluated for Polyneuropathies," *European Journal of Neurology* 14, no. 7 (July 2007): 788–792.

9. Y. M. Sun et al., "Opioids Protect against Substantia Nigra Cell Degeneration under Conditions of Iron Deprivation: A Mechanism of Possible Relevance to the Restless Legs Syndrome (RLS) and Parkinson's Disease," *Journal of the Neurological Sciences* 304, nos. 1–2 (May 2011): 93–101.

10. A. S. Walters et al., "Does the Endogenous Opiate System Play a Role in the Restless Legs Syndrome? A Pilot Post-Mortem Study," *Journal of the Neurological Sciences* 279, nos. 1–2 (April 2009): 62–65.

11. S. von Spiczak et al., "The Role of Opioids in Restless Legs Syndrome: An [11C] Diprenorphine PET Study," *Brain* 128, pt. 4 (April 2005): 906–917.

12. L. B. Weinstock and A. S. Walters, "Restless Legs Syndrome Is Associated with Irritable Bowel Syndrome and Small Intestinal Bacterial Overgrowth," *Sleep Medicine* 12, no. 6 (June 2011): 610–613.

13. M. Matsuo, "Restless Legs Syndrome: Association with Streptococcal or Mycoplasma Infection," *Pediatric Neurology* 31, no. 2 (August 2004): 119–121.

14. R. A. Franco et al., "The High Prevalence of Restless Legs Syndrome Symptoms in Liver Disease in an Academic-Based Hepatology Practice," *Journal of Clinical Sleep Medicine* 4, no. 1 (February 2008): 45–49; L. B. Weinstock et al., "Celiac Disease Is Associated with Restless Legs Syndrome," *Digestive Diseases and Sciences* 55, no. 6 (June 2010): 1667–1673; and L. B. Weinstock et al., "Crohn's Disease Is Associated with Restless Legs Syndrome," *Inflammatory Bowel Diseases* 16, no. 2 (February 2010): 275–279.

15. L. B. Weinstock et al. "Restless Legs Syndrome—Theoretical Roles of Inflammatory and Immune Mechanisms," *Sleep Medicine Review* 16, no. 4 (August 2012): 341–354.

16. C. J. Earley et al., "Altered Brain Iron Homeostasis and Dopaminergic Function in Restless Legs Syndrome (Willis-Ekbom Disease)," *Sleep Medicine* 15, no. 11 (November 2014): 1288–1301.

17. T. Ganz, "Hepcidin, a Key Regulator of Iron Metabolism and Mediator of Anemia of Inflammation," *Blood* 102, no. 3 (August 2003): 783–788; and F. Marques et al., "Altered Iron Metabolism Is Part of the Choroid Plexus Response to Peripheral Inflammation," *Endocrinology* 150, no. 6 (June 2009): 2822–2828.

18. Weinstock and Walters, "Restless Legs Syndrome Is Associated."

19. L. Ferini-Strambi et al., "The Relationship among Restless Legs Syndrome (Willis-Ekbom Disease), Hypertension, Cardiovascular Disease, and Cerebrovascular Disease," *Journal of Neurology* 261, no. 6 (June 2014): 1051–1068.

20. M. Hornyak et al., "What Treatment Works Best for Restless Legs Syndrome? Meta-analyses of Dopaminergic and Non-dopaminergic Medications," *Sleep Medicine Review* 18, no. 2 (April 2014): 153–164.

21. L. M. Trotti et al., "Iron for Restless Legs Syndrome," *Cochrane Database of Systematic Reviews* (May 2012): 5.

22. Weinstock et al., "Celiac Disease Is Associated."

23. C. Trenkwalder et al., "Prolonged Release Oxycodone-Naloxone for Treatment of Severe Restless Legs Syndrome after Failure of Previous Treatment: A Double-Blind, Randomised, Placebo-Controlled Trial with an Open-Label Extension," *The Lancet Neurology* 12, no. 12 (December 2013): 1141–1150.

24. J. Sobel et al., "Investigation of Multistate Foodborne Disease Outbreaks," *Public Health Reports* 117, no. 1 (January–February 2002): 8–19.

25. L. K. Turnbull et al., "Principles of Integrative Gastroenterology: Systemic Signs of Underlying Digestive Dysfunction and Disease," in *Integrative Gastroenterology*, ed. G. Mullen (New York, NY: Oxford University Press, 2011), 84–98.

26. E. Israeli et al., "Guillain-Barré Syndrome—A Classical Autoimmune Disease Triggered by Infection or Vaccination," *Clinical Reviews in Allergy & Immunology* 42, no. 2 (April 2012): 121–130.

27. L. B. Weinstock et al., "Restless Legs Syndrome in Patients with Irritable Bowel Syndrome: Response to Small Intestinal Bacterial Overgrowth Therapy," *Digestive Diseases and Sciences* 53, no. 5 (May 2008): 1252–1256.

28. L. B. Weinstock, "Antibiotic Therapy May Improve Idiopathic Restless Legs Syndrome: Prospective, Open-Label Pilot Study of Rifaximin, a Nonsystemic Antibiotic," *Sleep Medicine* 11, no. 4 (April 2010): 427.

29. L. B. Weinstock and S. Zeiss, "Rifaximin Antibiotic Treatment for Restless Legs Syndrome: A Double-Blind, Placebo-Controlled Study," *Sleep and Biological Rhythms* 10, no. 2 (April 2012): 145–153.

Chapter 7: Depression

1. As defined by the *Diagnostic and Statistical Manual of Mental Disorders*, 5th ed. (DSM-5) (Washington, DC: American Psychiatric Association, 2013).

2. G. W. Vogel et al., "Improvement of Depression by REM Sleep Deprivation: New Findings and a Theory," *Archives of General Psychiatry* 37, no. 3 (1980): 247–253.

3. R. Dantzer et al., "Inflammation-Associated Depression: From Serotonin to Kynurenine," *Psychoneuroendocrinology* 36, no. 3 (April 2011): 426–436.

4. J. Ross, *The Mood Cure: The 4-Step Program to Take Charge of Your Emotions—Today* (New York, NY: Penguin Books, 2003).

5. E. Jutkiewicz et al., "Behavioral and Neurobiological Effects of the Enkephalinase Inhibitor RB101 Relative to Its Antidepressant Effects," *European Journal of Pharmacology* 531, nos. 1–3 (February 2006): 151–159.

6. E. Jutkiewicz, "RB101-Mediated Protection of Endogenous Opioids: Potential Therapeutic Utility?," *CNS Drug Reviews* 13, no. 2 (Summer 2007): 192–205.

7. H. Zhang, "Endogenous Opioids Upregulate Brain-Derived Neurotrophic Factor mRNA through Delta- and Micro-Opioid Receptors Independent of Antidepressant-like Effects," *European Journal of Neuroscience* 23, no. 4 (February 2006): 984–994.

8. U. E. Lang and S. Borgwardt, "Molecular Mechanisms of Depression: Perspectives on New Treatment Strategies," *Cellular Physiology and Biochemistry* 31, no. 6 (2013): 761–777.

9. J. Phillips et al., "A Prospective, Longitudinal Study of the Effect of Remission on Cortical Thickness and Hippocampal Volume in Patients with Treatment-Resistant Depression," *International Journal of Neuropsychopharmacology* 18, no. 8 (March 2015).

10. T. Frodl, "BDNF Val66Met Genotype Interacts with Childhood Adversity and Influences the Formation of Hippocampal Subfields," *Human Brain Mapping* 35, no. 12 (December 2014): 5776–5783.

11. R. H. McCusker and K. W. Kelley, "Immune-Neural Connections: How the Immune System's Response to Infectious Agents Influences Behavior," *The Journal of Experimental Biology* 216 (January 2013): 84–98.

12. R. Dantzer and K. W. Kelley, "Twenty Years of Research on Cytokine-Induced Sickness Behavior," *Brain, Behavior, and Immunity* 21, no. 2 (February 2007): 153–160.

13. J. Younger et al., "The Use of Low-Dose Naltrexone (LDN) as a Novel Anti-inflammatory Treatment for Chronic Pain," *Clinical Rheumatology* 33, no. 4 (April 2014): 451–459.

14. A. J. Dean et al., "Does Naltrexone Treatment Lead to Depression? Findings from a Randomized Controlled Trial in Subjects with Opioid Dependence," *Journal of Psychiatry & Neuroscience* 31, no. 1 (January 2006): 38–45; and I. Petrakis et al., "Naltrexone and Disulfiram in Patients with Alcohol Dependence and Current Depression," *Journal of Clinical Psychopharmacology* 27, no. 2 (April 2007): 160–165.

15. A. J. Dean et al., "Does Naltrexone Treatment Lead."

16. American Psychiatric Association, *Diagnostic and Statistical Manual of Mental Disorders*, 5th ed. (DSM-5) (Washington, DC: American Psychiatric Association, 2013).

17. P. Tejedor-Real et al., "Involvement of Delta-Opioid Receptors in the Effects Induced by Endogenous Enkephalins on Learned Helplessness Model," *European Journal of Pharmacology* 354 (1998): 1–7.

18. P. Tejedor-Real et al., "Implication of Endogenous Opioid System in the Learned Helplessness Model of Depression," *Pharmacology Biochemistry and Behavior* 52, no. 1 (1995): 145–52.

19. S. Kent et al., "Sickness Behavior as a New Target for Drug Development," *Trends in Pharmacological Sciences* 13 (1992): 24–28.

20. N. A. Harrison et al., "Neural Origins of Human Sickness in Interoceptive Responses to Inflammation," *Biological Psychiatry* 66, no. 5 (2009): 415–422.

21. E. Miller, "Some Psychophysiological Studies of Motivation and of the Behavioural Effects of Illness," *Bulletin of the British Psychological Society* 17 (1964): 1–20.

22. L. Capuron et al., "Does Cytokine-Induced Depression Differ from Idiopathic Major Depression in Medically Healthy Individuals?," *Journal of Affective Disorders* 119, nos. 1–3 (December 2009): 181–185.

23. N. Müller et al., "The Cyclooxygenase-2 Inhibitor Celecoxib Has Therapeutic Effects in Major Depression: Results of a Double-Blind, Randomized, Placebo Controlled, Add-on Pilot Study to Reboxetine," *Molecular Psychiatry* 11, no. 7 (July 2006): 680–684.

24. R. J. Tynan et al., "A Comparative Examination of the Anti-inflammatory Effects of SSRI and SNRI Antidepressants on LPS Stimulated Microglia," *Brain, Behavior, and Immunity* 26, no. 3 (March 2012): 469–479.

25. S. Sacre et al., "Fluoxetine and Citalopram Exhibit Anti-inflammatory Activity in Human and Murine Models of Rheumatoid Arthritis and Inhibit Toll-Like Receptors," *Arthritis & Rheumatology* 62, no. 3 (March 2010): 683–693.

26. D. Bustamante et al., "Ethanol Induces Stronger Dopamine Release in Nucleus Accumbens (Shell) or Alcohol-Preferring (Bibulous) Than in Alcohol-Avoiding (Abstainer) Rats," *European Journal of Pharmacology* 591, nos. 1–3 (September 2008): 153–158.

27. D. J. Stein, "Depression, Anhedonia, and Psychomotor Symptoms: The Role of Dopaminergic Neurocircuitry," *CNS Spectrums* 13, no. 7 (July 2008): 561–565.

28. D. Bennabi et al., "Psychomotor Retardation in Depression: A Systematic Review of Diagnostic, Pathophysiologic, and Therapeutic Implications," *BioMed Research International* (2013). doi:10.1155/2013/158746.

29. C. Reuben, "CARA Model of Brain Repair at the Sacramento Drug Court," *Townsend Letter: The Examiner of Alternative Medicine*, January 5, 2007, http://www.townsendletter.com/Jan2007/CARA0107.htm.

30. S. S. Feinberg, "Combining Stimulants with Monoamine Oxidase Inhibitors: A Review of Uses and One Possible Additional Indication," *Journal of Clinical Psychiatry* 65, no. 11 (November 2004): 1520–1524.

31. D. L. Musselman et al., "Biology of Mood Disorders," in *Textbook of Psychopharmacology*, 2nd ed., ed. A. F. Schatzberg and C. B. Nemeroff (Washington, DC: American Psychiatric Press, 1998), 549–588.

32. D. Sasaki-Adams, "Serotonin-Dopamine Interactions in the Control of Conditioned Reinforcement and Motor Behavior," *Neuropsychopharmacology* 25, no. 3 (September 2001): 440–452.

33. P. Seeman, "Atypical Antipsychotics: Mechanism of Action," Canadian Journal of Psychiatry 47, no. 1 (February 2002): 27–38.

34. S. N. Blair et al., "Incremental Reduction of Serum Total Cholesterol and Low-Density Lipoprotein Cholesterol with the Addition of Plant Stanol Ester-Containing Spread to Statin Therapy," *American Journal of Cardiology* 86, no. 1 (July 2000): 46–52.

35. G. I. Papakostas, "Effect of Adjunctive L-Methylfolate 15 mg among Inadequate Responders to SSRIs in Depressed Patients Who Were Stratified by Biomarker Levels and Genotype: Results from a Randomized Clinical Trial," *Journal of Clinical Psychiatry* 75, no. 8 (August 2014): 855–863.

36. "Low-Dose Naltrexone for Depression Relapse and Recurrence," *Clinicaltrials.gov*, July 1, 2015, https://clinicaltrials.gov/ct2/show/NCT01874951.

Chapter 8: Autism Spectrum Disorder

1. J. Baio, "Prevalence of Autism Spectrum Disorder Among Children Aged 8 Years—Autism and Developmental Disabilities Monitoring Network, 11 Sites, United States, 2010," *Surveillance Summaries* 63, no. SS02 (March 2014): 1–21.

2. American Psychiatric Association, *Diagnostic and Statistical Manual of Mental Disorders*, 5th ed. (DSM-5) (Washington, DC: American Psychiatric Association, 2013).

3. G. O. Sallows and T. D. Graupner, "Intensive Behavioral Treatment for Children with Autism: Four-Year Outcome and Predictors," *American Journal of Mental Retardation* 110, no. 6 (November 2005): 417–438.

4. L. A. Vismara et al., "Can One Hour per Week of Therapy Lead to Lasting Changes in Young Children with Autism?," *Autism* 13, no. 1 (January 2009): 93–115.

5. G. H. Moody, "Interventions for Children with High Functioning Autism: A Review of Literature," *Master Moody*, January 2012, http://mastermoody.com/Master_Moody/Writings_files/LiteratureReview.pdf.

6. S. J. Rogers et al., "Autism Treatment in the First Year of Life: A Pilot Study of Infant Start, a Parent-Implemented Intervention for Symptomatic Infants," *Journal of Autism and Developmental Disorders* 44, no. 12 (December 2014): 2981–2995.

7. A. Ghanizadeh et al., "A Head-to-Head Comparison of Aripiprazole and Risperidone for Safety and Treating Autistic Disorders, a Randomized Double Blind Clinical Trial," *Child Psychiatry & Human Development* 45, no. 2 (2014): 185–192.

8. B. L. Handen et al., "Efficacy of Methylphenidate among Children with Autism and Symptoms of Attention-Deficit Hyperactivity Disorder," *Journal of Autism and Developmental Disorders* 30, no. 3 (June 2000): 245–255.

9. M. L. McPheeters et al., "A Systematic Review of Medical Treatments for Children with Autism Spectrum Disorders," *Pediatrics* 127, no. 5 (May 2011): 1312–1321.

10. L. Kanner, "Autistic Disturbances of Affective Contact," *Acta Paedopsychiatrica* 35, no. 4 (1968): 100–136.

11. B. Rimland, *Infantile Autism: The Syndrome and Its Implications for a Neural Theory of Behavior* (East Norwalk, CT: Appleton-Century-Crofts, 1964).

12. R. J. Hagerman et al., "An Analysis of Autism in Fifty Males with the Fragile X Syndrome," *American Journal of Medical Genetics* 23, nos. 1–2 (January–February 1986): 359–374.

13. B. Rimland et al., "The Effect of High Doses of Vitamin B6 on Autistic Children: A Double-Blind Crossover Study," *The American Journal of Psychiatry* 135, no. 4 (April 1978): 472–475.

14. D. J. Boullin et al., "Laboratory Predictions of Infantile Autism Based on 5-Hydroxytryptamine Efflux from Blood Platelets and Their Correlation with the Rimland E-2 Score," *Journal of Autism and Childhood Schizophrenia* 1, no. 1 (January 1971): 63–71.

15. B. Rimland, "Savant Capabilities of Autistic Children and Their Cognitive Implications," in *Cognitive Defects in the Development of Mental Illness*, ed. George Serban (Oxford: Bruner/Mazel, 1978), 43–65.

16. C. Gillberg and M. Coleman, *The Biology of the Autistic Syndromes* (London, UK: Mac Keith Press, 2000).

17. Ibid.

18. M. Herbert and K. Weintraub, *The Autism Revolution: Whole-Body Strategies for Making Life All It Can Be* (New York, NY: Ballantine Books, 2013).

19. K. L. Hyde et al., "Neuroanatomical Differences in Brain Areas Implicated in Perceptual and Other Core Features of Autism Revealed by Cortical Thickness Analysis and Voxel-Based Morphometry," *Human Brain Mapping* 31, no. 4 (April 2010): 556–566.

20. O. I. Lovaas, "Behavioral Treatment and Normal Educational and Intellectual Functioning in Young Autistic Children," *Journal of Consulting and Clinical Psychology* 55, no. 1 (February 1987): 3–9.

21. D. Granpeesheh et al., "Applied Behavior Analytic Interventions for Children with Autism: A Description and Review of Treatment Research," *Annals of Clinical Psychiatry* 21, no. 3 (July–September 2009): 162–173.

22. Lovaas, "Behavioral Treatment and Normal Educational."

23. S. M. Robertson, "Neurodiversity, Quality of Life, and Autistic Adults: Shifting Research and Professional Focuses onto Real-Life Challenges," *Home* 30, no. 1 (2010).

24. P. Howlin et al., "The Recognition of Autism in Children with Down Syndrome—Implications for Intervention and Some Speculations about Pathology," *Developmental Medicine & Child* Neurology 37, no. 5 (May 1995): 406–414.

25. C. R. Marshall and S. W. Scherer, "Detection and Characterization of Copy Number Variation in Autism Spectrum Disorder," *Methods in Molecular Biology* 838 (2012): 115–135.

26. J. E. Libbey et al., "Autistic Disorder and Viral Infections," *Journal of NeuroVirology* 11, no. 1 (February 2005): 1–10.

27. A. Vojdani et al., "Infections, Toxic Chemicals and Dietary Peptides Binding to Lymphocyte Receptors and Tissue Enzymes Are Major Instigators of Autoimmunity in Autism," *International Journal of Immunopathology and Pharmacology* 16, no. 3 (September–December 2003): 189–199.

28. P. Krakowiak et al., "Maternal Metabolic Conditions and Risk for Autism and Other Neurodevelopmental Disorders," *Pediatrics* 129, no. 5 (May 2012): 1121–1128.

29. E. J. Glasson et al., "Perinatal Factors and the Development of Autism: A Population Study," *Archives of General Psychiatry* 61, no. 6 (2004): 618–627.

30. G. Oliveira et al., "Mitochondrial Dysfunction in Autism Spectrum Disorders: A Population-Based Study," *Developmental Medicine & Child Neurology* 47, no. 3 (2005): 185–189.

31. J. J. Cannell, "Autism and Vitamin D," *Medical Hypotheses* 70, no. 4 (2008): 750–759.

32. D. L. Vargas et al., "Neuroglial Activation and Neuroinflammation in the Brain of Patients with Autism," *Annals of Neurology* 57, no. 1 (2005): 67–81.

33. A. Krigsman et al., "Clinical Presentation and Histologic Findings at Ileocolonoscopy in Children with Autistic Spectrum Disorder and Chronic Gastrointestinal Symptoms," *Autism Insights* 2 (2010): 1–11.

34. A. Angelidou et al., "Perinatal Stress, Brain Inflammation and Risk of Autism— Review and Proposal," *BMC Pediatrics* 12 (July 2012): 89.

35. M. Toichi and Y. Kamio, "Paradoxical Response to Mental Tasks in Autism," *Journal of Autism and Developmental Disorders* 33, no. 4 (August 2003): 417–426.

36. C. A. Pardo and C. G. Eberhart, "The Neurobiology of Autism," *Brain Pathology* 17, no. 4 (October 2007): 434–437.

37. S. J. James et al., "Metabolic Biomarkers of Increased Oxidative Stress and Impaired Methylation Capacity in Children with Autism," *The American Journal of Clinical Nutrition* 80, no. 6 (December 2004): 1611–1617.

38. M. G. Aman et al., "Prevalence and Patterns of Use of Psychoactive Medicines among Individuals with Autism in the Autism Society of Ohio," *Journal of Autism and Developmental Disorders* 33, no. 5 (October 2003): 527–534.

39. J. B. Adams et al., "Gastrointestinal Flora and Gastrointestinal Status in Children with Autism—Comparisons to Typical Children and Correlation with Autism Severity," *BMC Gastroenterology* 16 (March 2011): 11.

40. B. Rimland and S. M. Baker, "Brief Report: Alternative Approaches to the Development of Effective Treatments for Autism," *Journal of Autism and Developmental Disorders* 26, no. 2 (April 1996): 237–241.

41. A. Y. Hardan et al., "A Randomized Controlled Pilot Trial of Oral N-Acetylcysteine in Children with Autism," *Biological Psychiatry* 71, no. 11 (June 2012): 956–961.

42. P. A. Filipek et al., "Relative Carnitine Deficiency in Autism," *Journal of Autism and Developmental Disorders* 34, no. 6 (December 2004): 615–623.

43. S. J. James et al., "Metabolic Biomarkers of Increased Oxidative Stress and Impaired Methylation Capacity in Children with Autism," *The American Journal of Clinical Nutrition* 80, no. 6 (December 2004): 1611–1617.

44. W. Weber and S. Newmark, "Complementary and Alternative Medical Therapies for Attention-Deficit/Hyperactivity Disorder and Autism," *Pediatric Clinics of North America* 54, no. 6 (December 2007): 983–1006.

45. C. A. Sandman, "Beta-Endorphin Disregulation in Autistic and Self-Injurious Behavior: A Neurodevelopmental Hypothesis," *Synapse* 2, no. 3 (1988): 193–199.

46. C.A. Sandman, "Beta-Endorphin Disregulation in Autistic and Self-Injurious Behavior: A Neurodevelopment Hypothesis," *Synapse* 2, no. 3 (1988): 193–199.

47. M. Campbell et al., "Naltrexone in Autistic Children: An Acute Open Dose Range Tolerance Trial," *Journal of the American Academy of Child and Adolescent Psychiatry* 28, no. 2 (March 1989): 200–206.

48. M. Campbell et al., "Naltrexone in Autistic Children: A Double-Blind and Placebo-Controlled Study," *Psychopharmacology Bulletin* 26, no. 1 (1990): 130–135.

49. J. Panksepp et al., "Naltrexone and Other Potential New Pharmacological Treatments of Autism," *Brain Dysfunction* 4, no. 6 (January 1970): 281–300.

50. M. Campbell et al., "Naltrexone in Autistic Children: Behavioral Symptoms and Attentional Learning," *Journal of the American Academy of Child and Adolescent Psychiatry* 32, no. 6 (Nov. 1993): 1283–1291.

51. B. K. Kolmen et al., "Naltrexone in Young Autistic Children: A Double-Blind, Placebo-Controlled Crossover Study," *Journal of the American Academy of Child and Adolescent Psychiatry* 34, no. 2 (February 1995): 223–231.

52. M. P. Bouvard et al., "Low-Dose Naltrexone Effects on Plasma Chemistries and Clinical Symptoms in Autism: A Double-Blind, Placebo-Controlled Study," *Psychiatry Research* 58, no. 3 (October 1995): 191–201.

53. S. H. Willemsen-Swinkels, "Placebo-Controlled Acute Dosage Naltrexone Study in Young Autistic Children," *Psychiatry Research* 58, no. 3 (October 1995): 203–215.

54. R. Scifo et al., "Opioid-Immune Interactions in Autism: Behavioural and Immunological Assessment during a Double-Blind Treatment with Naltrexone," *Ann Ist Super Sanità* 32, no. 3 (1996): 351–359.

55. B. K. Kolmen et al., "Naltrexone in Young Autistic Children: Replication Study and Learning Measures," *Journal of the American Academy of Child and Adolescent Psychiatry* 36, no. 11 (November 1997): 1570–1578.

56. S. H. Willemsen-Swinkels, "The Effects of Chronic Naltrexone Treatment in Young Autistic Children: A Double-Blind Placebo-Controlled Crossover Study," *Biological Psychiatry* 39, no. 12 (June 1996): 1023–1031.

57. "Interview with Dr. Jaquelyn McCandless," Association for Comprehensive Neuropathy, June 19, 2009.

58. M. G. Chez et al., "Secretin and Autism: A Two-Part Clinical Investigation," *Journal of Autism and Developmental Disorders* 30, no. 2 (April 2000): 87–94.

59. H. Wei et al, "The Therapeutic Effect of Memantine through the Stimulation of Synapse Formation and Dendritic Spine Maturation in Autism and Fragile X Syndrome," *PLOS ONE* 7, no. 5 (2012).

60. J. Glenmullen, *Prozac Backlash: Overcoming the Dangers of Prozac, Zoloft, Paxil, and Other Antidepressants with Safe, Effective Alternatives* (New York, NY: Touchstone, 2001).

61. J. L. Benach et al., "A Microbial Association with Autism," *mBio* 3, no. 1 (February 2012); B. L. Williams et al., "Application of Novel PCR-Based Methods for Detection, Quantitation, and Phylogenic Characterization of *Sutterella* Species in Intestinal Biopsy Samples from Children with Autism and Gastrointestinal Disturbances," *mBio* 3, no. 1 (January 2012); and J. B. Adams et al., "Gastrointestinal Flora and Gastrointestinal Status in Children with Autism—Comparisons to Typical Children and Correlation with Autism Severity," *BMC Gastroenterology* 16 (March 2011): 11.

62. K. Horvath and J. A. Perman, "Autistic Disorder and Gastrointestinal Disease," *Current Opinion in Pediatrics* 14, no. 5 (October 2002): 583–587; and J. W. Critchfield et al., "The Potential Role of Probiotics in the Management of Childhood Autism Spectrum Disorders," *Gastroenterology Research and Practice* (2011).

63. T. C. Theoharides, "Is a Subtype of Autism an Allergy of the Brain?," *Clinical Therapeutics* 35, no. 5 (May 2013): 584–591.

64. A. Angelidou, "Neurotensin Is Increased in Serum of Young Children with Autistic Disorder," *Journal of Neuroinflammation* 7 (August 2010): 48.

65. R. Scifo et al., "Opioid-Immune Interactions in Autism: Behavioural and Immunological Assessment during a Double-Blind Treatment with Naltrexone," *Ann Ist Super Sanita* 32, no. 3 (1996): 351–359.

66. "Interview with Dr. Jaquelyn McCandless."

Chapter 9: Cancer

1. B. M. Berkson et al., "Revisiting the ALA/N (Alpha-Lipoic Acid/Low-Dose Naltrexone) Protocol for People with Metastatic and Nonmetastatic Pancreatic Cancer: A Report of 3 New Cases," *Integrative Cancer Therapies* 8, no. 4 (December 2009): 416–422; and B. M. Berkson et al., "Reversal of Signs and Symptoms of a B-Cell Lymphoma in a Patient Using Only Low-Dose Naltrexone," *Integrative Cancer Therapies* 6, no. 3 (September 2007): 293–296.

2. I. S. Zagon and P. J. McLaughlin, "Naltrexone Modulates Tumor Response in Mice with Neuroblastoma," *Science* 221, no. 4611 (August 1983): 671–673.

3. H. Sobel and G. Bonorris, "Effect of Morphine on Rats Bearing Walker Carcinosarcoma 256," *Nature* 196 (December 1962): 896–897.

4. P. Sacerdote, "Opioids and the Immune System," *Palliative Medicine* 20 (January 2006): 9–15.

5. S. Elmore, "Apoptosis: A Review of Programmed Cell Death," *Toxicologic Pathology* 35, no. 4 (2007): 495–516.

6. S. D. Meriney et al., "Morphine-Induced Delay of Normal Cell Death in the Avian Ciliary Ganglion," *Science* 228, no. 4706 (June 1985): 1451–1453.

7. M. S. Kim, "Protective Effects of Morphine in Peroxynitrite-Induced Apoptosis of Primary Rat Neonatal Astrocytes: Potential Involvement of G Protein and

Phosphatidylinositol 3-Kinase (PI3 Kinase)," *Biochemical Pharmacology* 67, no. 7 (April 2001): 779–786.

8. I. Tegeder and G. Geisslinger, "Opioids as Modulators of Cell Death and Survival—Unravelling Mechanisms and Revealing New Indications," *Pharmacological Reviews* 56, no. 3 (September 2004): 351–369; B. Afsharimani et al., "Morphine and Tumor Growth and Metastasis," *Cancer and Metastasis Reviews* 30, no. 2 (June 2011): 225–238; K. Gach et al., "The Role of Morphine in Regulation of Cancer Cell Growth," *Naunyn-Schmiedeberg's Archives of Pharmacology* 384, no. 3 (September 2011): 221–230; and S. Bimonte et al., "The Role of Morphine in Animal Models of Human Cancer: Does Morphine Promote or Inhibit the Tumor Growth?," *BioMed Research International* (2013): 1–4.

9. K. Gach et al., "Opioid-Receptor Gene Expression and Localization in Cancer Cells," *Central European Journal of Biology* 6, no. 1 (February 2011): 10–15.

10. M. Ishikawa et al., "Enhancement of Tumor Growth by Morphine and Its Possible Mechanism in Mice," *Biological & Pharmaceutical Bulletin* 16, no. 8 (August 1993): 762–766.

11. J. W. Boland, "Effects of Opioids on Immunologic Parameters That Are Relevant to Anti-tumour Immune Potential in Patients with Cancer: A Systematic Literature Review," *British Journal of Cancer* 111, no. 5 (August 2014): 866–873.

12. L. Koodie et al., "Morphine Inhibits Migration of Tumor-Infiltrating Leukocytes and Suppresses Angiogenesis Associated with Tumor Growth in Mice," *The American Journal of Pathology* 184, no. 4 (April 2014): 1073–1084.

13. T. Reisine and G. I. Bell, "Molecular Biology of Opioid Receptors," *Trends in Neurosciences* 16, no. 12 (December 1993): 506–510.

14. G. W. Pasternak and X. Y. Pan, "Mu Opioids and Their Receptors: Evolution of a Concept," *Pharmacological Reviews* 65, no. 4 (September 2013): 1257–1317.

15. R. Al-Hasani and M. R. Bruchas, "Molecular Mechanisms of Opioid Receptor-Dependent Signalling and Behavior," *Anesthesiology* 115. No. 6 (December 2011): 1363–1381.

16. R. J. Lefkowitz and S. K. Shenoy, "Transduction of Receptor Signals by Beta-Arrestins," *Science* 308 no. 5721 (April 2005): 512–517.

17. L. M. Luttrell et al., "Activation and Targeting of Extracellular Signal-Regulated Kinases by Beta-Arrestin Scaffolds," *Proceedings of the National Academy of Sciences U.S.A.* 98 no. 5 (February 2001): 2449–2454.

18. P. H. McDonald et al., "Beta-Arrestin 2: A Receptor-Regulated MAPK Scaffold for the Activation of JNK3," *Science* 290, no. 5496 (November 2000): 1574–1577.

19. E. M. Unterwald et al., "Quantitative Immunolocalization of Mu Opioid Receptors: Regulation by Naltrexone," *Neuroscience* 85, no. 3 (August 1998): 897–905.

20. E. M. Unterwald et al., "Chronic Opioid Antagonist Administration Upregulates Mu Opioid Receptor Binding without Altering Mu Opioid Receptor mRNA Levels," *Molecular Brain Research* 33, no. 2 (November 1995): 351–355.

21. A. Tempel et al., "Antagonist-Induced Opiate Receptor Upregulation in Cultures of Fetal Mouse Spinal Cord-Ganglion Explants," *Brain Research* 390, no. 2 (March 1986): 287–291.

22. V. A. Alvarez et al., "Mu-Opioid Receptors: Ligand-Dependent Activation of Potassium Conductance, Desensitization, and Internalization," *Journal of Neuroscience* 22, no. 13 (July 2002): 5769–5776.

23. M. Navarro et al., "Functional Interaction between Opioid and Cannabinoid Receptors in Drug Self-Administration," *Journal of Neuroscience* 21, no. 14 (July 2001): 5344–5350.

24. T. Rubino et al., "Long-Term Treatment with SR141716A, the CB1 Receptor Antagonist, Influences Morphine Withdrawal Syndrome," *Life Sciences* 66, no. 22 (April 2000): 2213–2219.

25. A. Hotzoglou et al., "Morphine Cross-Reacts with Somatostatin Receptor SSTR2 in the T47D Human Breast Cancer Cell Line and Decreases Cell Growth," *Cancer Research* 55, no. 23 (December 1995): 5632–5636.

26. I. S. Zagon and P. J. McLaughlin, "Naltrexone Modulates Tumor Response in Mice with Neuroblastoma," *Science* 221, no. 4611 (August 1983): 671–673.

27. R. N. Donahue et al., "Low-Dose Naltrexone Targets the Opioid Growth Factor-Opioid Growth Factor Receptor Pathway to Inhibit Cell Proliferation: Mechanistic Evidence from a Tissue Culture Model," *Experimental Biology and Medicine (Maywood)* 236, no. 9 (September 2011): 1036–1050.

28. M. Adams et al., "The Anti-proliferative Effect of Lenalidomide on MM Cells in Vitro Is Ameliorated by Prior Exposure to Pomalidomide, and Agent with Activity against Lenalidmode Resistant MM Cells," *ASH Annual Meeting* (2009): 4926.

CONTRIBUTORS

Dr. Jill Cottel

Dr. Jill Cottel is native to Southern California and grew up in San Diego. She received her bachelor's degree with honors at University of California at San Diego (UCSD) in biochemistry and cell biology. She received her medical degree from UCSD School of Medicine. She is board certified in internal medicine and is a diplomate of the American Board of Holistic Integrative Medicine. She has twenty years of internal medicine experience and is currently in private practice in Poway, California.

Dr. Angus G. Dalgleish

Dr. Angus G. Dalgleish trained at University College Hospital, where he earned an intercalated degree in anatomy with Professor J. Z. Young. Following house jobs, he took a position with the Royal Flying Doctor Service of Australia for one year and stayed on to train in internal medicine and oncology at hospitals in Brisbane and Sydney. He returned to the United Kingdom in 1984 and undertook a thesis on retroviruses with Robert Weiss. He was then appointed as senior clinical scientist at the MRC Clinical Research Centre in Northwick Park, London, where he pursued his interests in HIV pathogenesis and the potential of thalidomide to treat chronic diseases. His suggestion that analogs of thalidomide could lead to enhancement of therapeutic activity and reduction of side effects was co-opted by David Stirling of Celgene, and this partnership led to the licensing of Revlimid (lenalidomide) and Pomalyst (pomalidomide) for myeloma and lymphoma. He was awarded the Joshua Lederberg Award in 2011 in recognition of this work.

Since 1991 he has been professor of oncology at St. George's, University of London. During this time he has focused on the immunotherapy of cancer and has conducted numerous clinical trials involving a variety of vaccines and immunotherapy. Since 2001 he has been the principal of the Cancer Vaccine Institute, currently focusing on the revival of the mycobacterium-based vaccines that were dropped by SR Pharma and now resurrected by Immodulon Therapeutics. He is on numerous scientific advisory boards involving the development of vaccines and immunotherapy, including Celgene, Immodulon, CureVac, and Bionor Pharma. He was chief investigator of a randomized clinical trial in patients with metastatic pancreatic cancer for Immodulon that tested IMM-101 and gemcitabine versus gemcitabine alone, which has shown a significant survival advantage for the IMM-101 combination with no significant toxicities. These findings were presented in early 2015. In addition, his observations that Revlimid is co-stimulatory when given with vaccines has been confirmed in a randomized study of a therapeutic vaccine for HIV, where it significantly increased the CD4 counts that have not responded to HAART or the vaccine alone.

J. Stephen Dickson

Stephen Dickson is a pharmacist who has worked in the LDN field for ten years, dealing with in excess of ten thousand patients in this decade. He has been involved in primary research into LDN mechanisms of action and still closely works with most UK LDN prescribers to make sure patients have a safe and effective treatment regimen. Stephen is the 2013 winner of the Royal Pharmaceutical Society Awards "Leader in Pharmacy" designation. He spends most of his time working within the National Health Service and is superintendent of five pharmacies, which means that he provides advice on safety and clinical questions to the pharmacists he works with.

Stephen says he "got involved in LDN a while back" and has been an advocate of the therapy since very early on. "I had a friend with a really low immune cell count; no one knew why it was happening. The doctors had tried everything they could think of to get it back up, to no avail—so I suggested she try LDN. Remarkably, two weeks after starting the LDN her cell count was within normal range," he said. Although that example does not exactly concern multiple sclerosis, Stephen says the example proved to him the clinical efficacy.

"It definitely does something—and if people are benefiting from LDN therapy, then why not try? It is a lot less harmful than many of the other drugs used to treat MS. Just don't take it when you are on opiates, and check with your doctor or pharmacist first!

"We fully support the trials that are getting underway—the faster we get double-blind, placebo-controlled studies, the faster everyone can get LDN on the NHS!"

Stephen is currently renovating an old house, running a church youth group, and is also starting a new business using fingerprint technology to safely identify patients. Stephen said, "Basically, in my spare time, I sleep!" He can be reached via superintendent@dicksonchemist.co.uk or http:// www.dicksonchemist.co.uk.

Dr. Kent Holtorf

Kent Holtorf is the medical director of the Holtorf Medical Group and the nationwide Holtorf Medical Group Affiliate Centers. He is also founder and director of the nonprofit National Academy of Hypothyroidism (NAH), which is dedicated to dissemination of new information to doctors and patients on the diagnosis and treatment of hypothyroidism.

He has personally trained numerous physicians across the country in the use of bioidentical hormones, hypothyroidism, complex endocrine dysfunction, and innovative treatments of chronic fatigue syndrome, weight loss, fibromyalgia, and chronic infectious diseases including Lyme disease.

He is a fellowship lecturer for the American Academy of Anti-Aging Medicine, the endocrinology expert for AOL Health, and a guest editor and peer-reviewer for a number of medical journals, including *Endocrine*, *Postgraduate Medicine*, and *Pharmacy Practice*. Dr. Holtorf has published a number of peer-reviewed endocrine reviews, including on the safety and efficacy of bioidentical hormones, inaccuracies of standard thyroid testing, testosterone replacement for men and women, the diagnosis and treatment of growth hormone deficiency, the diagnosis and treatment of adrenal dysfunction in chronic fatigue syndrome and fibromyalgia, peripheral thyroid hormone conversion and its impact on TSH and metabolic activity, and the clinical applications of thyroid hormone transport into cellular tissue.

He has helped to demonstrate that much of the long-held dogma in endocrinology is inaccurate. He is a contributing author to Denis Wilson's just published *Evidenced-Based Approach to Restoring Thyroid Health*.

Dr. Holtorf has been a featured guest on numerous TV networks and TV and radio shows such as CNBC, ABC News, CNN, EXTRA TV, Discovery Health, The Learning Channel, *The Today Show*, *The Dr. Dean Edell Radio*

Program, The Glenn Beck Radio Program, Nancy Grace, Fox Business, ESPN, *The Rush Limbaugh Show, CBS Sunday Morning, The Sean Hannity Show,* and So Cal News. He has been quoted in numerous print media, including *The Wall Street Journal, Los Angeles Times, U.S. News & World Report, San Francisco Chronicle,* WebMD, *Health, Elle, Better Homes and Gardens, Us Weekly, Forbes, Cosmopolitan, New York Daily News,* and *Self,* among many others.

Dr. Skip Lenz

Dr. Skip Lenz received his B.S. in pharmacy from Massachusetts College of Pharmacy in 1973. He conducted advanced studies in qualitative/ quantitative analysis at Harvard University. Skip spent two years at Brown University studying statistical analysis. He studied advanced pharmacology at Florida Atlantic University. From 1989 through 1992 he entered an MS/ PhD program in gerontology at Nova Southeastern University. He received his doctorate in 1999 at University of Florida School of Pharmacy with a special interest in patient compliance. He has been a fellow of the American Society of Consultant Pharmacists for over twenty years. He was named a fellow in the American College of Veterinary Pharmacists in 2004. Over the last decade he was a speaker at over two hundred conferences, including on topics such as low dose naltrexone, legal issues in pharmacy for dispensing practitioners, animal pharmacology, and the appropriate use of transder- mals, as well as many topics in pharmacology and the law.

Dr. Wai M. Liu

Dr. Wai M. Liu obtained his PhD in Medical Oncology from St. Bartholomew's Hospital in London, and has been actively involved in cancer research for over 20 years. His work has focused on tackling cancer by formulating new treatment strategies for pre-existing drugs that exploit unique combina- tion regimens, as well as developing novel anticancer compounds. He has shown how tumors treated with certain drugs respond by communicating in different ways with cells of the immune system. Tumor cells are able to produce bioactive substances that impact upon dendritic cell and T-cell responses, and he showed that chemotherapies can negate these pro- cancerous effects, which provides an exploitable route into a novel strategy for attacking cancer.

Dr. Liu has also been instrumental in the development of cannabinoids as a putative anticancer agent and was the first to describe a therapeutic benefit of combining this class of drug with irradiation to treat brain cancer. His work is recognised internationally and has been regarded by many as helping to get the compound recognised as a possible medicine by US organizations. He has been a guest speaker on a number of broadcasts, such as the BBC and ITV. He has also been interviewed on numerous occasions in print media such as *The Independent, Daily Mail, The Times, Wall Street Journal,* and *The Washington Times.*

Dr. Mark H. Mandel

Dr. Mark H. Mandel is a pharmacist who specializes in bioidentical hormone replacement therapy (BHRT); weight loss and management; pain management; and the treatment of chronic health conditions with an integration of conventional care, adjunctive therapies, and natural pharmaceutical alternatives. He is the owner and president of Mark Drugs Roselle, a compounding pharmacy located in west suburban Roselle, Illinois, the first PCAB-accredited compounding pharmacy in the state. Mark is a graduate of the University of Illinois College of Pharmacy and Midwestern University College of Pharmacy in Downers Grove, Illinois. He is cohost of the weekly radio health show *The Doctor and the Pharmacist,* which airs on Saturday mornings on AM 1160. Mark speaks regularly to physicians, pharmacists, and nursing and community groups, providing insights on how natural pharmaceutical alternatives and prescription compounding can enhance patient care and quality of life. Mark believes in approaching patient care from a "ground up" point of view that rejects traditional medicine because it tends to treat chronic illnesses with a reactive approach versus a proactive one that addresses the real source of the problem. Mark believes that many chronic health conditions such as rheumatoid arthritis, hypertension, high cholesterol, obesity, insulin resistance and diabetes, and intestinal and gastric problems can be treated and potentially eliminated with combinations of natural pharmaceutical alternatives that are easy to use, safe, and effective.

Mark lives in Schaumburg, Illinois, with Sarah, his wife of over thirty years. They have three daughters, Rachel, Rebecca, and Shannon.

Trisha L. Myers

Trisha L. Myers is a recent graduate of Saint Louis University, where she received a master's of medical science in physician assistant studies. She is board-certified and has chosen to specialize in gastroenterology. She received a bachelor's of science, summa cum laude, from Truman State University, where she studied health science and biology. She is interested in the relationship between the many conditions that occur subsequent to and/or are exacerbated by small intestinal bacterial overgrowth and the ensuing systemic inflammation. A native St. Louisan, she lives there with her family, who all share a great love for the St. Louis Cardinals.

Julia Schopick

Julia Schopick is the author of the Amazon-bestselling book *Honest Medicine: Effective, Time-Tested, Inexpensive Treatments for Life-Threatening Diseases.* Through her writing, her website (http://www.HonestMedicine.com), and her radio interviews, Julia's goal is to educate people about little-known but promising treatments their doctors may not know about. One of the treatments Julia is most passionate about is LDN. She also enjoys making presentations to large groups, both in person and remotely, via Skype.

Dr. Mark Shukhman

Dr. Mark Shukhman, MD, is a psychiatrist in private practice in the suburbs of Chicago. Prior to becoming an MD, his interests included alternative medicine and mathematics. Dr. Shukhman's practice is focused on such problems as mood, anxiety, sleep, sex, appetite control, memory problems, chronic pain, and addiction to opioids and alcohol. Dr. Shukhman is frequently consulted on psychosomatic problems and psychiatric symptoms that accompany general medical conditions. His treatment approach is based on neuropsychiatric interpretation of symptomatology and usually consists of combination of medications with vitamins, supplements, and reflexotherapy. LDN is a part of his psychopharmacological armamentarium for treatment of mood disorders, eating disorders, and addictions.

Dr. Shukhman teaches, including as a "doctor teaching other doctors." He was on the faculty of a board preparation course, advisory panels, and multiple grand rounds. He has also served as a primary investigator for several pharmaceutical research studies.

Rebecca Shukhman

Rebecca Shukhman is a student at Midwestern University's Chicago College of Osteopathic Medicine. She is a research assistant at Associates in Psychiatric Wellness, LP. Her previous research experience with the CAN (cognitive and affective neuroscience) lab was related to studying the brains of the "superagers"—elderly individuals with statistically better-preserved cognitive functioning.

Dr. Jill P. Smith

Dr. Jill Smith is board-certified in internal medicine and gastroenterology; a professor in the Department of Medicine at Georgetown University in Washington, DC; professor emeritus at the College of Medicine of Pennsylvania State University; and the director of Clinical & Translational Research, LLC. Dr. Smith has been first or senior author in over eighty publications in peer-reviewed medical or scientific journals and has received many honors and awards including distinction as president from the American Pancreatic Association; Physician of the Year from Health Care Heroes in Pennsylvania; Alpha Omega Alpha from the Medical Honor Society; the College of Medicine mentoring award; and the Sullivan Pancreatic Cancer Research Endowment Chair, to name a few.

Dr. Smith's passion is to take innovative ideas and discoveries from the laboratory and apply them to patient care vis-à-vis drug development and target-specific therapy. She enjoys being a triple-threat physician in academic medicine, where she is involved in research, teaching, and patient care. Dr. Smith says her goal is to improve survival from cancer and chronic illnesses while improving quality of life.

Dr. Brian D. Udell

Dr. Brian D. Udell, MD, is a leader in the health care industry, with over thirty-six years of experience. Presently, he practices special needs pediatric medicine in Davie, Florida, focusing on children with developmental disabilities including ADHD and autism.

Dr. Udell is involved in several professional health care and charitable organizations and has received numerous honors and awards. He holds a BA from Temple University, an MD from Thomas Jefferson University, and an MBA from the University of Miami.

Dr. Udell says, "I was the first pediatrician to publish medical research regarding the use of computers to calculate and document infant intravenous nutritional support. With my partners in Pediatrix Medical Group, we were able to expand treatment to infants throughout the US, providing a new, improved level of in-hospital care for high-risk newborns.

"This newly emerging epidemic of attention deficit and autism spectrum disorders has inspired me to focus my training and practice on problems with childhood development. Because there has been such an explosion of families who are affected by these challenges, I am in a unique position to help evaluate all of the available research and treatments, and to provide a combination of all of the proposed therapies so that my patients have the best chance to achieve their highest potential."

Dr. Udell publishes information about this unique practice at his popular website http://www.TheAutismDoctor.com.

Dr. Leonard B. Weinstock

Dr. Weinstock is board-certified in gastroenterology and internal medicine and is president of Specialists in Gastroenterology and the Advanced Endoscopy Center. Dr. Weinstock teaches at Barnes-Jewish Hospital, is an associate professor of clinical medicine and surgery at Washington University School of Medicine, and is a primary investigator at the Sundance Research Center. Dr. Weinstock received a BA magna cum laude from University of Vermont and an MD from University of Rochester School of Medicine. He completed his postgraduate training and was chief resident in internal medicine at Rochester General Hospital. His gastroenterology fellowship was performed at Washington University School of Medicine.

Dr. Weinstock is an active lecturer and has published more than eighty articles, abstracts, editorials, and book chapters. He is currently researching the role and treatment of small intestinal bacterial overgrowth, dysbiosis, and systemic inflammation in restless legs syndrome, irritable bowel syndrome, complex regional pain syndrome, Ehlers-Danlos syndrome, fibromyalgia syndrome, chronic pelvic pain syndrome, and rosacea. He is very interested in colon cancer prevention and has expertise in colon cancer screening and advanced polypectomy techniques. Further information is available at http://www.gidoctor.net.

Dr. Deanna Windham

Dr. Deanna Windham is a graduate of Oklahoma State University College of Osteopathic Medicine. She completed her internship at Brooklyn Hospital and her residency in family practice at Chino Valley Medical Center, California. She has devoted her medical career to training in and practicing integrative medicine, which involves using all scientifically proven modes of medical treatment and disease prevention as opposed to using solely the Western medicine approach. She is a fellow in the Anti-Aging and Regenerative Medicine Program through the Florida State University College of Medicine and the American Academy of Anti-Aging Medicine. She is a nationally respected integrative physician, lecturer, and author. She works at Whitaker Wellness Institute, the largest integrative medical treatment center in the country, where she is the director of quality assurance and the medical safety director of the Hyperbaric Oxygen Department. She has lectured nationally and given interviews on varied topics in integrative or holistic medicine. She is a prolific writer, having published several articles on various subjects and authored dozens of patient informational handouts. She also enjoys coauthoring science fiction and fantasy novels with her writer husband. They live blissfully unaware of the real world as the parents of two delightful young princesses and an imperial cat in southern California.

INDEX

Note: page numbers followed by f or t refer to Figures or Tables

ABOUT THE EDITOR

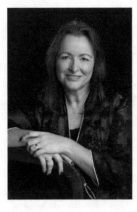

Photo by Julia Holland

Linda Elsegood is the founder of the LDN Research Trust, which was set up in the UK as a Registered Charity in 2004, and is the editor of *The LDN Book*. Diagnosed with MS in August of 2000, she started LDN therapy in December of 2003, and now has a better quality of life and hope for the future. Through the Trust, she has connected thousands of patients, doctors, and pharmacists around the world with information, articles, and patient stories about LDN.

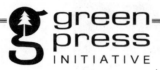

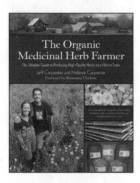
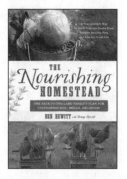
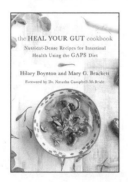
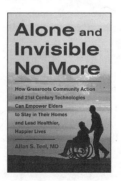
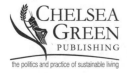

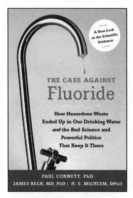
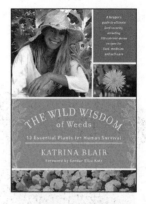
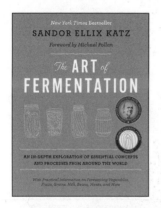
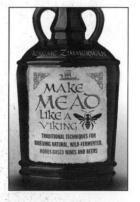
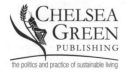